AGING GRACEFULLY

DR. YOGITA

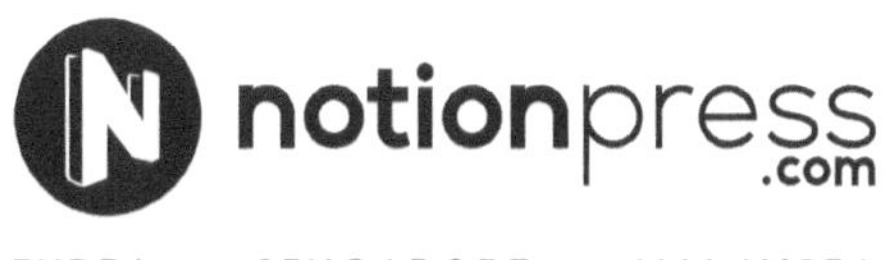

notionpress.com

INDIA • SINGAPORE • MALAYSIA

Notion Press Media Pvt Ltd

No. 50, Chettiyar Agaram Main Road,
Vanagaram, Chennai, Tamil Nadu – 600 095

First Published by Notion Press 2021
Copyright © Dr. Yogita 2021
All Rights Reserved.

ISBN

Domestic 978-1-63940-399-8
International 978-1-68509-763-9

Contents

Acknowledgement

Foremost by the grace of God, I would like to thank my father with whom at this age as well I can dig on depth in intense subjects.

Along want to express my gratitude truly to my mother who indeed conveyed me the merits of being women.

My sincere appreciation is for my husband and my kids-Nikunj and Ritisha, who served as a stimulus in successfully accomplishing the process.

I am thankful to my significant other- my mother-in-law, my brothers and sis-in-laws, Eshan, who always pat on my back even for my smallest achievement.

I thank Nikhil and Akshay for neatly putting together their artistic elements of art in sketching of images.

I finally want to thank all enthusiast who always kept me on toes in savouring the fitness journey.

I am grateful to the reputed publishing house-Notion, for our tie up.

Dr Yogita

Fight or Flight

Attempting to understand what make life meaningful, by that it can help us to lead a better life for us has a lot of answers because every person has different understanding towards life. For me, life is meaningful when you have a purpose, coherent with your values and significant to express who you are.

Among the widespread ideologies to keep me motivated what would work best other than "Work is Worship" quoted by Gandhiji which justifies the significance of work in our life and our attitude towards it. In his view any work (Karma) done with dedication and passion in their respective fields, although may be small deserve praise or reward that is equivalent to worship (Puja). In this effort I was worthy in the habit to shield my karma by efficiently making a good connect of homemaker and working woman.

Lockdown was the time of threats for humans and left its mark on us deep down. Although those were the bad times where the need was to put everything in right perspective without losing your brain, it can be an opportunity to refresh your appetite, your desire.

This is what this alteration did, it took hold of me and lift a step ahead in a row for worship from the narrow confines of my individualistic concerns to share the general responsibility for the broader concerns of humanity, as far as women is concerned, putting little bits of good whenever and wherever possible to lead the way to her physical, mental, psychological and social happiness which ultimately balance the state of her body, mind and soul.

Sitting empty out of the blue, on the spur of the moment my mind laid my eyes comprehensively on my body, deep down the core and the flow went uninterrupted into a closed prolonged succession. My soul scuffled for idle away much of life's time in waste, consequently fetching to this physical state of mine progressively worst.

It's been rightly said that adversity and loss make a man wise. In this sense from the recollection of my past it made me wise to take over the responsibility for the future. Rather than looking back on years gone by, I may begin scrambling to prioritise and accomplish better health in the second half of my life, before all else. From my half-unfinished knowledge to get there I will have to push myself because why somebody else do something for me? no one else is going to do it for me, therefore I started to go just more than skin deep.

In the battle of life while keep on fighting with daily chores, busy schedules and more, woman surrender her healthy living. Even if she desires, how do she make sure that her body is healthy? as health awareness and health care needs are not well understood, acknowledged with lack of availability of resources, which is why a big question has been created for the well being of woman world-wide. The WHO affirms that today woman's health has become an urgent priority and to achieve optimum healthcare outcomes shows necessity to initiate a range of activities and strategies ensuring they have access to quality care of her health.

Where such a big crisis and purpose stands, for which a lot can be done, I did not find it appropriate to procrastinate the urgency, as I too believe in 'Giving While Living' when if not money, you can actively devote your skills and time to make a difference sooner rather than later. That's why for the manifestation of my goal, without delay, before "Giving" for better living, I honored my intuition to invest in myself first, before all else. Investing to take full knowledge of one's body and act accordingly, can give you good interest.

During this time, I was most keenly interested in knowing the preconceptions about aging, whose roots are deep. I trailed right from the anatomy, physiology of the human body to various theories of aging and its aesthetic aspects, and found that the stage through which I'm going today is due to its effect, which is natural but, in time it has not been handled could lead to sufferings. It made me to admit that we all change and a mid life crisis is evidence which could come as psychological change in the form of depression, social change compelled by the youth obsessed society or physical change which usually over the years appear as weight gain, shrinks, sagging skin ,hair loss, etc.

After carefully weighing the reasons, I thought the foremost choice I could make is to somewhat alleviate the physical changes which in succession could treat their psychosocial ailments.

As you can see- at my age start trying things to see if they work demands great exertion, but my open mind has a reservoir of law of possibility who never make a deficit to try more things as it is more likely that one of them will work for me. And yes! making a place for 'workouts' in my daily chores begin obliged me to feel and look good.

When I was at home, I retrospected myself that when I'm not having any physical access to patients, what best I could do to reach them? Also the thought 'Giving While Living' enlightened me to go virtually for promotion of health and disease prevention among women through educating them. Sometimes the smallest step in the right direction ends up being the biggest step in your life, and if that step is for the well being of women, wouldn't that be outstanding? For the life of me I will be so pleased that I'd taken that one small step.

I conceived, live at home, there can be a deal for the benefit of woman, so that is 'exercises', as of today, is one of the best way to prevent diseases and keep your ticker strong. If you can't do it too, do something every day to get moving by walking, jogging, swimming or dancing. Those who want to further boost their metabolism, build muscles and maintain strong bones, they can combine strength training along with cardio.

I think one or the other women must be finding in the same circumstances as I'm in, are likewise apprehensive as well, but were deficient in getting the right way. So, eventually after getting quite self-assured and seeing some welcome changes in me, I obviously by all odds start to alley myself to them, to vocalise with them, addressing them and what come into being-some considered me, some had a passionate debate, somewhere participants experience brought about some open suggestions ushering insight and creative solutions while some were waiting for the storm. Their curiosity could bring about a lead to step forward and bestow a strong arm in the throes of depression.

The questions I struggled with, this question will likewise be in the minds of my readers, so I would like to share some of my conversation.

I don't have any time for exercise, forget me.

Me: Dear, you are the master of your own time means while staying energised, you can certainly get more things done better while you enjoy.

I gave up exercises as I couldn't find results in 3–4 months.

Me: It's good, at least you had made a choice for workouts and remember, every choice take us closer to the target. Also, believe me there are nothing stronger than those two: patience and time, if you could continue they will do it all.

Why to choose for exercise at this age, when life is still on?

Me: Look, with age we become sedentary, there are many reasons, and if we have to keep fit in this age than active lifestyle becomes important.

Physical health benefits of exercise, in a way it maintains or loose weight, reduces the impact of illness and chronic disease, enhance your mobility, flexibility and balance also benefitting your mental health, are no more hidden from us. If you make a choice to daily add my mere some inclusions in intelligible ways, it will pay its cost in a way you can to some extent sustain some age related changes whereas bound to take its course. So, act in time.

I often delay todays workouts on tomorrow.

Me: Remember, lost time is never found again, we can't keep todays hour for tomorrow. Whatever you are meant to do, do it now. The conditions are always impossible.

I spent hours in gym, but couldn't get the desired result.

Me: Don't forget the hours you have spent either in gym or at home for those are useful in the sense that has value or you can call it your "investment" not an expense.

A subject professor said me-

Can I start at this age for I lost my much past?

Me: Don't hold your past, madam. You cannot turn the clocks but can do your best to make tomorrow a happier time.

For I knew happiness lies in the joy of achievement, to make it come true, my initial goal was to awake every avid exerciser early in the morning while not stressing on any of home work.

With available resources I set my goal balancing my time. Aside from giving lessons and workout plans in a manner corresponding to my knowledge, I also got cognisant of life and mind too. By learning new things with interest and enthusiasm, I entered new phase of life and my circle broadened.

I must say, I was lucky to join curious women supporting 'Jungian theory' that holds life is a key to individuation process of self-actualisation and self awareness that contain many potential paradoxes, and digging dipper the crisis was associated with awareness of aging.

These concerns kept me on toes to formulate the path of graceful aging by safeguarding positive mindset in this mid life turmoil, to some extent most of the time doesn't need professional help, except when you see distressing symptom that impair your functioning, for e.g.a thyroid or diabetic condition, arthritis, previous major surgeries may cause many changes, seek professional help.

Opening new doors and doing new things for healthier life, leading the way to destination the road was not straight, challenges started coming the way, bombarding of messages, mails never let me to sit idle, but with attitude and constantly striving to give my best effort, eventually overcoming the problems.

While getting rendezvous with woman's, I felt like everyone is waiting from the long time expecting for me to get the bottom of their curiosity that was in view of half knowledge which is dangerous, and fear to achieve it escorted by lot of ignorance.

To achieve my goal outside the comfort zone, I directed my efforts towards giving them knowledge and make them into action, in which I started getting success. This was limited to just one group, what about those who are waiting, will anyone show them the way to tighten up their worries? Here showed me the only way- 'to write a book'.

Now I had to adopt the mindset of an author. What is expected of you and the message you have to give, also underline all that in a book; this efficiency meant the fortune teller of my book.

Here you could see the worries and concerns which I have embraced appealing as chapters, have been hit to me at different times and predominantly forewarning physical concerns about aging killing your looks, I found only after going in depth about it. For the ease of reading, I whipped them into shape serially from head to toe.

Here, the title image I put through, take you closer to the vulnerable area of your body and on engaging those areas in workouts, how it looks is also been told. It may happen to come to you in varying degree. Also these concern in your body don't come alone, it may be in an amalgamation of many and with different facets. But to spot the exact problem I highlighted the only area at a time. The labour I put in drawing images of workout is merely based on my vision for looking towards it, and only some part of it is pictured, in my estimation after reading you too can visualise the actual techniques and act along.

In the beginning my style of composition writing was laid like a prescription, every time it started to look petrified, devoid of life. To make it possible for the women to be seen that this situation is not just mine it is theirs too, also to make a good connect with her, furthermore she can also relate her story to me and can prepare herself as much as she can like me- I added my stories.

This is how my story went from a sudden thought entering in my head and reaching a book in your hand, keeping the reader centric perspective in mind where I bestow a simple message towards empowering others to make a change in her life.

Wherefore I Caught the Pulse of Aging Facet

The world at large is inclined for comprehensive and disease liberated life. Me, you and also the last person in life, want to live life. And if to this hypothesis, health supports then there is meaning to live this life. Conversely, the body is grinding to one side, on that, raging of disease, seems like before life ends everything is over.

Me at this age, worry about life ahead. But how judicious is to worry about things happening in the future. Today what I have in hand, I can ride it. In this day itself, the reflection of me is inscribed.

The women of my period who are in the middle of life, somewhere mind and body getting tired, it is understanding, and now somewhere on looking at the body they are worried to see its decline. The various anguish in the body, feeling stiffness of the body with that; seems like her work capacity is decreasing now. I own empathy as a companion. But tell the truth, if today we foresee this and grid our lions, so tomorrow your body will substantiate or not. let's cherish the body with this hope.

In this regard, the structure of this body, in that, the changes happening with age, on that score I got curious to get information. Upon it, the present state of my body would be able to decide her intended favoured position and decline.

Like your nature your body is also intricate. Even after giving so many theories the mystery of aging is maintained. But still we do not stop questioning these mysteries lurking right around the corner. Each one of us have to do is face them-differently.

Its usual you get nerve wracking about aging when you abruptly see wrinkles and grey hairs. This is an outward display of age, with this there are persistent and perpetual changes in your body like your heart, bones, muscles, joints, digestive system, bladder and urinary tract, eyes and ears, skin, weight, memory and thinking skill, it even has an impinge on your sexuality. I reaffirmed myself by practicing hard the scientific and difficult fact that aging is inevitable and intrinsic. Now it's crucial to understand the process which from head to toe makes an impact, but we anyhow live this 'age', despite that don't want to understand it.

Our aging body at one hand, follows the genes who are designed for scheduled maintenance, repair and defence the systems who are responsible for its maintenance, controls the hormones for the ease of aging, also holds immunity against getting vulnerable to infectious diseases and thus aging and death; on the other hand, it combat environmental damages by wearing and tear of cells, holding damage made by free radicles, slowing down the cross linked protein damages done to cells and tissues. All this process goes on microscopically undetected inside the body. We get its suffix from some notations, like some women notice an increase in changing of body shape with age, their lower body is not in commensuration with upper body, their belly, thighs, hips start to appear disfigured. Many women also notice an increase in belly fat as they get older, even they aren't gaining weight. This is likely due to decreasing level of oestrogen, which appears to influence where fat is distributed in the body.

While in some it has come into view, in this time of life, they start becoming more sedentary, life style changes come to your lives and in some there is lack of physical activity. As well in this phase your muscle mass and muscle strength is going to fall short. Thus your primary aging, environment, obesity, disease, either distinct or combiningly effects the muscular skeletal system, the very first. And depending on the magnitude of aging in the muscle skeletal system, further impact your quality and length of life.

If you want to get rid of these dilemmas, empower this system, is the only primary thought. Concentrating on this system I explore about body muscles, its origin and insertion, their activities related to the bones and joints and studied the speciality of there physiology.

Inside, a human being is said to have so many skins covering the depths of the heart when from outside, its actually has the skin covering the skeletal muscles, synergically responsible for moving the external parts of the body and the limbs. The way these muscles hugs the skeleton, gives it a curvy shape and tone, I'm in its Love, and strong envious desire for such an aesthetic physique lasts forever. The way by my facial muscles minutely helps my countenance to curl up my lips, frown my forehead, and even the way to miem my words, mask my face, wink my eyes to add expressions, I love it.

Glorified knowledge of muscular system, surely the thought of keeping it for the handle is touching the mind. If you get apprehensive while reading this, as I myself was, even then, keep your faith on top of the fear, because if we start removing small-small stones then big mountain too can be removed. Everything you want is on the other side of fear and as there are far, far better things ahead than any we leave behind.

I understood while reading that fortunately those loses can be made or partially it can be overcome or at least significantly delayed by consciously adding some well-established counter measures against aging and ought to be emphasised as part of lifestyle essential to healthy living. It illustrated me, what else would work better to resist the fall, other than ensuring eat healthy and exercise often. Now, let food be thy medicine and exercise be a magic potion which allow your muscles to repair, replicate the muscle cells, form new muscle protein strands and allow blood oxygen to circulate quicker the whole body.

My story like this, started by doubting on me, to which wonderfully equipped science finally responded. It elucidated me the sources for upholding my body and conveyed the effective way to live healthy and fit- that was exercise.

If you find any of its benefits, I believe you would find countless ready-made facts and figures of its pertinent applicability, from your internet to magazines and where not. But some authentic information so that you understand my curiosity to write a book, also by keeping mindful of its advantages you could have tendency to exercise on her own, in the wake of this I need to write.

On continuing full body workouts, women cranked up sharing few of her immediate personal worries to me personally, which was seen to create a sense of numbness in them. I caught their pulse and altered my teaching and writing perspective, as well.

In your youth you don't have to please anyone as long as your physique makes it all the point, but with increasing age the spotlight fades away, the reason for this in some evidence is poor lack of muscle proportion and body measurements of your body, and therefore it does not pleases your eyes. In consequence you may have to face the hardships submitted further.

You will see in it, the worries and concerns which I mentioned as chapters, mainly any muscle characteristic of your aesthetic group of muscles is affected which superfluous incommensurate your physique with age. Therefore in the form of compound exercise I have bestowed you many ways of exercise to overcome, like-bench press, shoulder press, pull up, chin up, deadlift, squat, leg press. With all, the smaller muscles that are usually ignored, which has unique distinct importance in making of physique; something to active them too, like-bicep curls, tricep curls, chest fly, leg extension, hamstring curl, calf raise.

With your upper and lower splits to accentuate your facial aesthetic, muscle work is necessary to ride them too. likewise also worked on them predominantly and included some face lift exercises.

By not loosing the sight of the fact, by enticing their wants, when I created and implemented my workout program, so touched the heart of women. May be it touch your heart too.

Just Starting Out in the Field of Workout?

If you are a neophyte, take your pair of shoes and start walking at a comfortable pace outside or indoors on the terrace, so your body gets into gear to perform at least for three days a week and gradually progress by adding two or more moves or days.

Further begin with 35 minutes endurance training by cycling, brisk walking, running, swimming or can go for treadmill, stationary cycle, rowing machine.

Further increase your speed and incline by finding a hill to tackle and decrease back to baseline, reducing your speed, incline and resistance.

Total body strength for beginners

Once you start your cardio regularly, from that day forward you will automatically wish to move beyond that. When the awareness of the body increases, you will sigh for some new appraisals on your own one's initiative. To each of the muscle group, considering their usefulness, would you like to train. In order that you have to make a routine for the next week on two non-consecutive days of the week.

In the first place start with 5–10 minutes of cardio or some warm up sets of each exercise. On the condition that, no work is done on two days in a row at the same muscle groups, so, one day the upper body and the other day the lower body, divide the exercise in this way. After a few weeks you can modify sets or repetitions. Primitively, your body's own resistance is enough, to further tighten your body, it is expected to challenge your body hard, it requires equipment. The equipment I described (pushup bar, dumbbells, kettle bell, resistance band) in whomsoever workout, use them.

In the beginning supervise by yourself, do not make haste, first go for 1 set of 8–12 repetitions. Raise ahead to 2–3 sets. Don't forget to make provision for 30 seconds or one minute break between each workout.

In preference to just burning calories for being healthy and fit, our body needs stretching, too, owing to the fact that flexible muscles allow your joints to move through a full range of motion, mitigates the risk of injury, reduces muscle soreness and improve posture, releases excess muscle tension, aids in pain free movements, promotes muscle repair.

In the last to maximise the benefits of exercise concentrate on exercise specific breathing. While doing your running or jumping jacks you probably breaths in through mouth but nose is the preferred way to get oxygenated and when intensity ramps up, through the mouth. Here follow consistent breathing.

Remember the rule of cannon for strength training- inhale while relaxation and exhale during exertion. During your abdominal exercises you probably stop breathing as you crunch your body then also keep breathing. While squatting inhale when you begin to lower down and exhale as you come to the starting position. During pushup inhale while lowering your elbows down to the ground and exhale as you come back to the start.

You apprehend the initiative to start workout, it's a benediction, do one more thing, if you have any health problems like heart disease, kidney disease or type 1 or 2 diabetes, don't hesitate to consult your doctor. If you take advice in time you can implement your workout plan with safety measures and in a better way.

Pro-Workout, Embellish Your Home Gym

You must be suspecting why all around a volcano of health and fitness has erupted though this accusation is groundless, think for yourself, the pursuit for which our body is made for, are we able to do it in a substantial way in this changing lifestyle? Workouts are therefore seen as an "alternative lifestyle" with the aim to do justice to the body.

Your workouts, you can do every day like walking, jogging, skipping, swimming or if your goal is to either gain muscle or weight loss, for these states, you need weight training. Don't think that I'm recommending a gym sculpt figure for you; I'm advising you have an expected body fit. For each of your muscle group to train, I resorted many chapters. To do these workouts you can own your resistance or some resistance can also be given with equipment.

This too the opinion of many people, physical fitness can be found by going to the gym......I have been endeavouring, while staying indoors, you can eventually embrace gym-like perquisite, using time vantage and at relatively low cost. And in this long time of lockdown, when we are locked in the house, there is a reason why we should look for the alternative of gym at home itself.

You have enough space where you can keep one matt, your equipment and where some pilates you could do it smoothly. Then that place be the corner of your bedroom, covered terrace, or let it be the space below your staircase. You cushion that place, install organiser to keep equipment, long mirror can also be installed.

Many ladies consider a treadmill sufficient, seeing this it costs a lot of money you can also use one jump rope as a cardio. Would be appropriate instead one gym weight lifting multipurpose fitness bench which is adjustable where you can incline, decline, flat and can be used in almost any exercise.

In addition, buy a single kettle bell, pair of adjustable dump bells (an entire set of dumbbells), a set of resistance bands which give you the same muscle toning in the absence of heavy fixtures. Moreover make use of your simple towel for stretching as it is also a good way to improve flexibility in the muscle groups.

Make sure that you take few moments around each workout for doing roller press/massage the major muscles using 'foam roller' which is a simple cylinder, light weight, handy, occupies less space and prevents imbalances and overuse injuries.

Be mindful of the fact that during workouts you loose body fluid through sweat. Hence it's expected to drink enough fluids to maintain your body temperature and performance, before and during workouts. Also, you need to rehydrate after each session, for that drink more fluid than you lost while exercising. Sole water is elite in overcoming your fluid loss. Ergo forearm yourself to carry enough water before workouts.

Keep Moving

Life is about accepting the challenges along the way, choosing to keep moving forward and savouring the journey. If you have willingness to carry then age is just a number. No matter what your age is, what physical restrictions you have, at what level your fitness is and what for you want to make a change weather its for weight loss, to get healthy or for hourglass figure, take up the gauntlet in transit and ascend.

Once you psych yourself up for compliance with act and schedule your approximate each type of exercise around the week, good luck starts coming your way.

You see, no two days are alike, if any day you feel disappointed, lack of motivation, don't endure it, rather take out this page number and read my 'keep moving' paragraph, it will all set fire your belly necessary to seek your goal.

While talking to women, tells me for they are in the idea of starting an exercise, some also do commit me, but this is just one aspect. What I truly want is actually "starting" your workout which is completely a different ball game.

If someday in the morning, your body tells you're a little too sore, I tell u, its normal when you try new activities and this doesn't mean you should stop workouts which most of the ladies do in haste, instead you do it regularly or often it will be into your habit; this soreness will automatically get away.

In some case I received, they were dissatisfied saying that on the way to workout, next day they were not able to move, it's because they were carried out in excess and there is a need to withdraw next workout. Without a doubt mistakes will be made, but isn't it nice to think that tomorrow is a new day with no mistakes in it yet?

At the leading edge don't compare yourself with someone else's version of thin. Accepting yourself burns the most calories.

Plan for Healthy Diet

The word diet is used in two perspective, one- the kind of food a person is having constantly or regularly, and second- a special course/ item of food to which a person restricts themselves, either to loose weight or for medical reasons. For me aforesaid 'diet' means 'healthy diet'. That's because 'healthy diet' and 'diet for weight management' are often related, as both promote healthy weight management. Therefore, from the beginning we should aim healthy diet who has different types of food in certain quantities and proportions, in which carbohydrates, proteins, fats, vitamins and alternative nutrients through-and-through fulfils our requisite.

While thinking of 'diet' you have to begin at the end of your comfort zone and your willingness to work for them. Purpose of healthy diet, taken for today and not tomorrow, does not happen like this. You have to proactively make a long term lifestyle change not a momentary change. Also, a healthy diet compliments your workout program. If you spik and span your diet and exercise regularly, you can hope for your weight to make it on its own.

But, if you choose to loose weight or build muscles, it's impossible to do without a goal specific meal plan which would get the desired effect. Here are others, and me too do not advocate a single specific diet plan because only one unequivocal plan could not work for all. Here I think, who can be your dietician better than you? Considering this take some time to sit down and formulate a balanced diet to benefit your whole body and according to your choice, lifestyle, adjust your macro and micro nutrients.

If you are working out from 2 to 5 days a week lesser than 30 minutes, you will not be burning many calories and that being the case you need not to increase your calorie intake. Instead fix simply on healthy eating-getting right amount of proteins, grains, vegetables and fruits throughout the day. The food structure for Indians is such that their everyday meals contains enough macro and micronutrients less in evidence for their food. Due to this those who do moderate exercise, need not to very a lot for their everyday needs are meet. Fast food culture is also confined here, many believe on traditional foods which is succeeding through generations but with changing work culture their is a need to alter somewhat in terms of quantities and meal timings either.

On the other hand, if you are working out harder and longer either to lose weight, build muscle or keep up your fine, tuned body, it's imperative to have a goal-specific meal plan to obtain the best results.

what- ifs to loose weight?

In a bouts of weight loss, I see the point that some suddenly starts humming a tune of weight loss and adopt frivolous ways. Some straight away take a plunge into HIIT/resistance training such as weight lifting which is injudicious; practically its founded that those who fought with a regular start of low intensity training definitely reduced weight while reducing stress.

Such ladies also force themselves to restrict on diet. In a hurry to reduce weight, while exaggerating exercises begins to starve themselves. Hold dear, best things can be done between these extremes. Moderation is the answer. Instead of giving up, corroborate your dietary regimen with adequate proteins, fats, carbohydrates. Daily fix of lean proteins such as egg white, poultry, lean meat or pulses preserves lean mass while dieting phase. Continue to have fibre rich carbohydrates in low to moderate quantity such as oats, potatoes, rice and whole grains. Don't set aside fats from your diets, right kind of essential fatty acids are essential for cell membrane, hormone production, improves your body composition, mental and physical performance.

What-ifs to gain weight/muscle mass?

Daily servings of proteins, from animal or plant sources, hoists protein synthesis for muscle building and keep the amino acid concentration in the blood constantly high helping muscles to repair, thus fulfilling the needs of high proteins after exercises and during regeneration.

Notably add mighty complex carbohydrates like whole grain products, potatoes, rice, which are processed slowly keeping blood sugar levels stable and supply the body with energy long term but avoid simple carbohydrates like sugar, fruit juices.

Frequently asked questions-what are the foods that should be taken pre-workout and post-workout?

To fill up your energy pool you need to constant recharge for giving enough energy before and after workout. A pre-workout meal should consist mainly of complex carbohydrates and partial proteins, about 1 hour before your workout. After your workout, you have to be sharp-witted to provide sufficient supply mainly of proteins and fast carbohydrates within 30 minutes to prevent nutritional deficiencies and loss of muscle mass.

Remember, your diet plan will be working only if your digestive system be well.

If it's not, then you can suffer from digestive diseases, constipation and obesity. In such conditions only exercises won't work. While taking meals, without getting stuck in screens, give full attention to your food with a focused mind that's because the relation between mind and body. If you will eat with heart, your digestive enzymes will secrete properly who will digest your food well. Also, if you suffer from any digestive ailments, get cured first.

Pertaining to diet habits and cravings are seen as the common enemy which builds barrier that needs to be broken down otherwise every time they knock, you can't help but let them in. No one of us left, whatever their habits, not addicted to and are very well aware of its domination.

Think this through for a second and evaluate those habits of yours. Think- do they empower you, limit you or help you form reaching goal or disempower you, free you or hinder you. Remake your habits.

Craving is another powerful desire to which some are encouraged to get addicted and so we crave more, it may be your physical appetite or emotional need. While controlling your craving if you feel deprived and gets desire for spicing some taste during the week you can eat certainly anything you want in any of the day of week.

A day can really slip when you're deliberately avoiding what you are supposed to eat. Avoid hunger pangs and set your day with breakfast, lunch, dinner and some evening snacks.

Receding Hairline

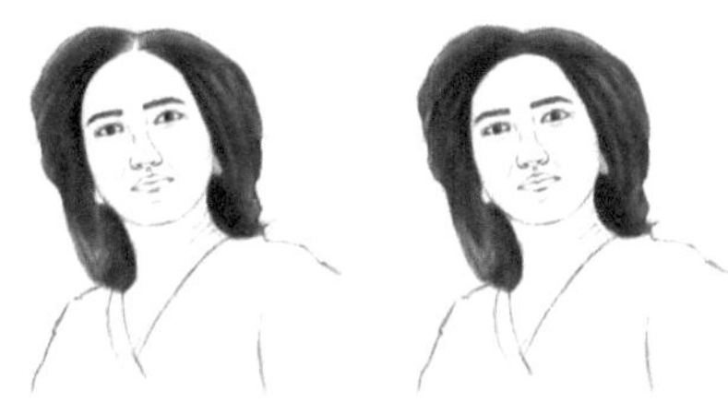

"Hey hey women! What's been happening?" I'm right here! with you throughout, taking you to my amazing world of self actualisation by endearing self-esteem impacted by aging.

In want of change, let's celebrate the above distinction between the images.

There has been a land on which we stand, another land is that under which we have complete existence, that top notch is- a land of head. This land also has the potential to produce, nearly 100,000 hair follicles are below this land which grows hairs and develop them. But your hormones, emotional health and age gets overshadowed and these reducing its land, slowing down its beauty, and barrenness in some is more likely.

Although your hairline configure and explicate your face, which seems to me rarely straight across due to lateral mounds, widows peak and concavities which is inevitable at any time and any state of life.

One person's hairline is 'matchless" than another in size and height, and its also 'fearless', in the sense that sometimes with age this stops growing the hairs in one or both temples and shapes her "M' or ride straight back horizontally exposing your forehead.

How would you recognise your receding hairline?

After going through this page, some are getting cognisant of hairline for the first time as she is not enlightened with the alteration of age and if have, then aren't decisive for herself. Not too hard to understand. If you see your forehead appears longer than 2 to 2.4 inches or 5 to 6 cm above the eyebrow (labella) then its out of ordinary and it would be phenomenal to prefer lowering your hairline or let your doctor tell you the type of hair loss you are experiencing by performing a "pull test", blood test to look for thyroid or any other scalp infection causing hair loss.

The gradual progression of hairline expose your forehead, are linked with the rise of fortunes, which enthral Indian women. Todays aristocrat knows, fate doesn't rise like that, it has to be made, and prepares their mind to conquer fortune. She is understanding the impact of receding hairline on the beauty of her face and emotional disturbing is also happening.

The signs of exact hair loss is not from regular shredding, rather meets you with hair thinning on your temples. Men and women, receding hairline are spotted in both of these. But genes does not annoy you as much as it does to men. It doesn't fall you victim to 'bald spots', but by thinning your hair reduces their volume.

In one case, none of your generation can stay away from it, however you can try to find the option and in another kind women often take offence on themselves by scraping back hairstyles, you can also get rid out of them. But on stoping the molecular change that occur with age, whole world is eyeing the scientists. Thanks to science, on its progress, remedies and alterations will be displayed soon, we hope, until the later time can depend only on our elbow grease.

While studying the muscles(frontal) below for scalp; it was found that it has no hand in receding hairline. So, its needless to build it. But there is a need to relax this. Because this muscle gets tensed with neck muscles while working in the desk, which further lead to headache. This being the case, mechanical stimulation of the scalp by massage is significant to relax, with which the blood circulation of the scalp increases which furthermore into the bargain work on reducing the hair fall.

When I read how to take action so as to be free of this, for a spell I got fascinated by the ways of "regrowth" of hairs set forth by medical field of aesthetics and anti-aging. But do our hair need that much? as much as to some life-threatening conditions.

For ever, relying on some medicines, you even thought to undo it, so you have to be prepared for the side effects as well.

Custom of our rich culture seem ridiculous but yet scientific. By touching the feet of the elders (it is also decent if you touch yours), blood flow reverts and increases blood circulation in all parts of the body especially head, also stimulates pituitary gland which controls growth and development.

These customs are analogous to todays 'science of inversion' where their fundamentals and goal match, the only distinctive method is that you have to massage the scalp with warm oil and do your head upside down for total 4 minutes, for a week or unless you want.

Or get to the any position as below, aiming your head below your heart. If discomfort or dizziness persists, immediately halt.

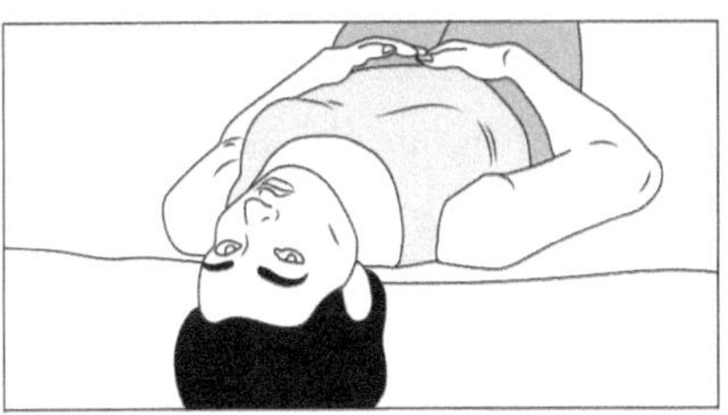
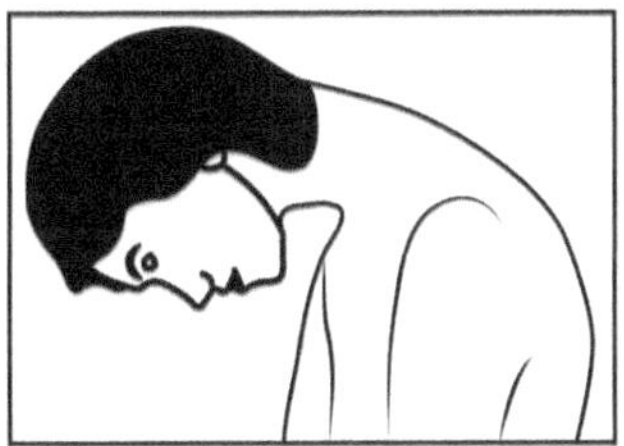
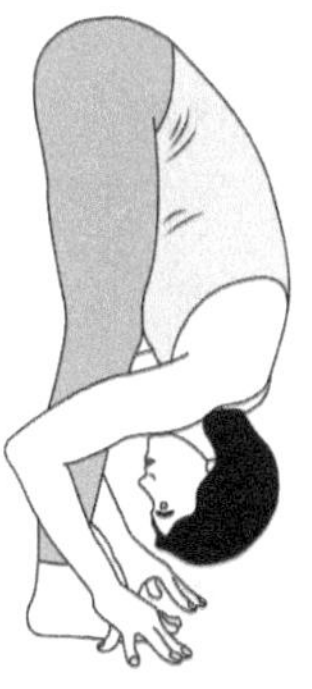
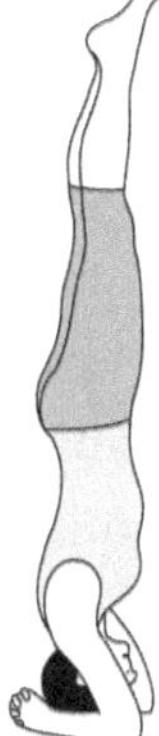

"chasing angels or fleeing demons, go to the mountains"

Each one of us "go" to the mountain has their own reasons and mine saying this "Chasing blood circulation or fleeing hair loss, make mountain of your body" has its own reasons, in the sense that it allows gravity to enhance blood circulation till the endest cell of head and beats hairloss. You may need to practice this version of the pose for a long time until your body starts to loosen up more to work with regards to straightening the legs while upholding a long spine.

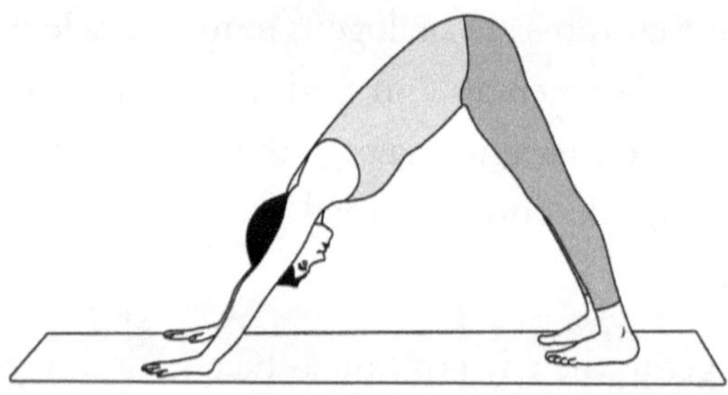

As stated "it's in the roots not the branches, that the trees greatest strength lies" in like manner the strength of the hair is also located in their roots, thereby it easily tolerate the assault of aging, thyroid, hot rods, relaxing and straightening chemicals. For now, if the roots of the hairs get proper nutrition like trees, so they won't fall weak. Remember getting awareness to nutrition filled diet is a first step towards any change.

You know who is no. 8 in periodic table and no.1 in existence? I would say that, this present misfortune must have made you aware of this, very well. Yes! this is oxygen. We disregarded it, nature immediately informed us how close we are to death.

This pandemic has taught us to check blood oxygen levels, now oxygen who is the center of our life process, which goes to each cell of our body and nurtures it, also practice increasing its level. For this what would be better than respiratory exercises and some walking? Gradual in succession your hairline will also get auspicious signs of this exercise.

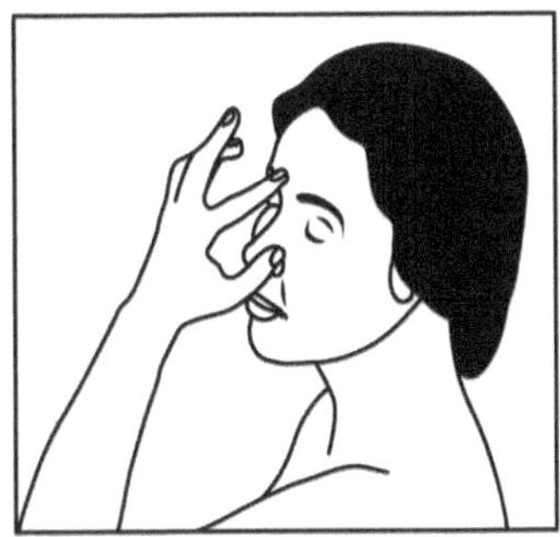

As much as you spent on your external beautification, many more less than that, you to your body costs to get strengthen from within.

Just to tickle your belly I tell you only one exercise. Recall the journey of your hair from where you were born bald.

Forehead Wrinkles

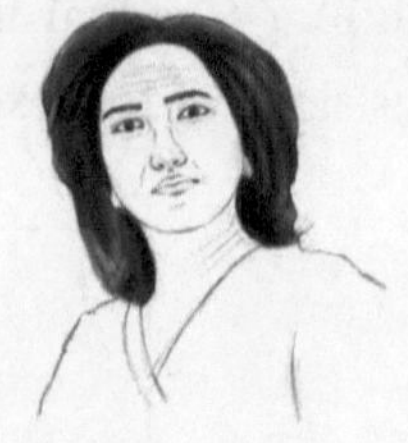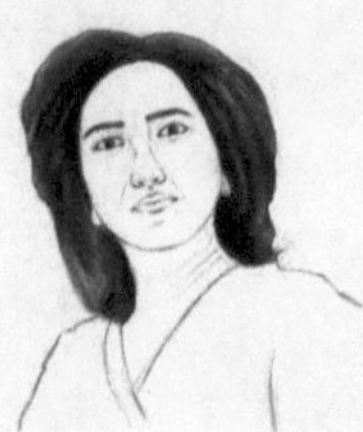

Forehead is distinct as it accentuates human brain for their solitary potential of imagination and the divine center for spiritual markings of Hindus customs in India, each having a definite significance. For eg.-the red bindi (dot) on forehead indicates woman's potent energy and has an understanding that its where the growing strength in women lies, not the forearm. On top of that, forehead confirms the real love of a man who can thrill it by kissing.

This high esteemed place as well withstands the cycle of time appearing as wrinkles. Forehead winkles as it may dishearten you, but are nobody to growl. With age the muscles that created the lines to begin with the first place get concrete with loss of collagen. It's obvious that staring into screens, stress, gravity, pollution, behavioural habits, genetics and the corrugated muscle can also cause frown lines or "the 11s" (deep vertical lines) on the forehead.

It is not certain when you can guess you will have wrinkles. In your time of life between 20 and 30, is the good age while your skin inherently turnout less supple and further brittle, undergo lesser making of natural oils and fails to keep fat in the deep skin layers, encouraging more striking lines. Also in winter of life, eye muscles becomes progressively worse to this degree that when we make eyes to open, we are likely to use forehead muscles or eyebrow muscles of nearby vicinity. Its then becomes vital to strengthen forehead frontal muscles and orbicularis oculi muscles of eye in order to minimise their appearance as you cant literally make wrinkles to banish.

If you want to guard the array of your face and lift your skin elasticity and little resistant, train yourself to do everything you fear to loose.

Start the order with face warm up. To start with squeeze and release eyelids, stare in an angry or fierce way, loosen up your face, make smiles, gently squeeze your face between your fingers, thereafter pat your face with wet warm cloth and relax.

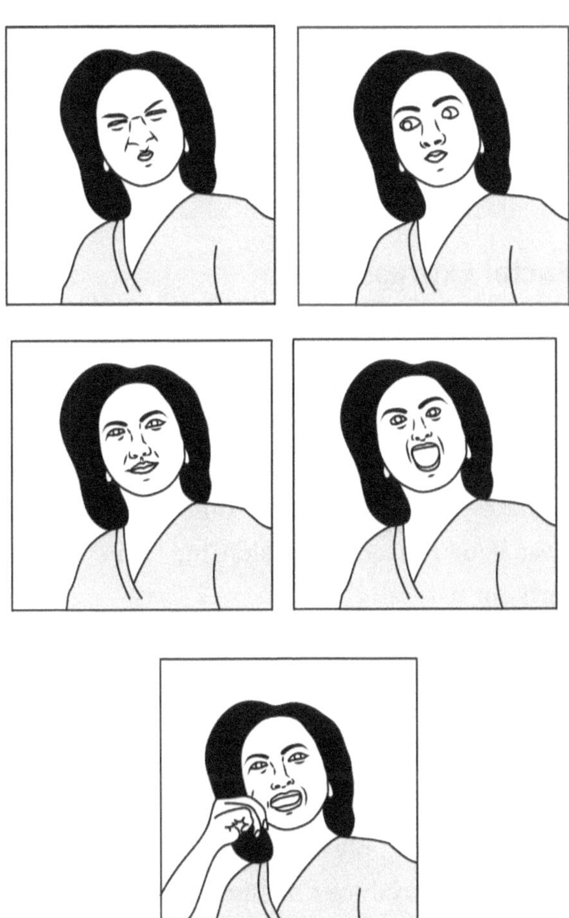

Rubber

This exercise helps to remove horizontal lines on forehead and should be done smoothly with constant breathing while doing.

Wrap your hands behind and put them on the boarder of your hairline on the forehead. Pull your hands back, little. Purse your lips with "O" and look down. Hold for few seconds and feel the tension on the forehead. Repeat for 10–20 times.

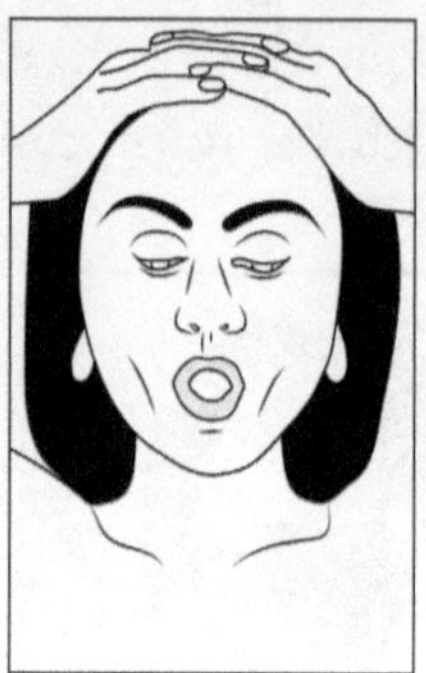

Facial Expressions

Basic facial expression of emotion is universal. We know that also for the effective communication, appropriate facial expressions are important, but some female have the habit of making unusual excessive facial activity. If I tell you these could accentuate facial wrinkles, would you make some move to control it? If yes, then, wear your relaxed expression for hours and subsequently it will turn out natural.

Massage

Massage with little oil by firmly applying pressure from the centre of the temples towards outward with the fingers for 15–20 times.

You can also apply aloe vera pulp which contains malic acid, discovered to reduce fine lines by tightening and toning the skin, or by simply running your fingers up and down on the forehead activates muscles tissues and blood flow, relieves tension around eyebrows, thereby reducing lines.

Brow Ptosis

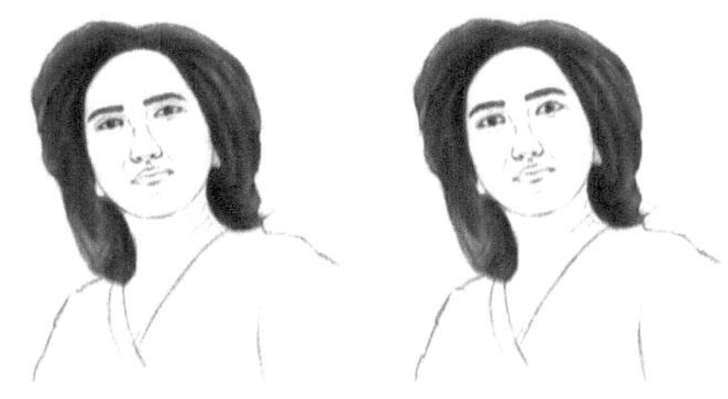

Retrospect your face shape, your eyebrows silhouette configuration is determined by the face shape. Finical eyebrows make a significance whether you appear tired or fresh as daisy. The nick of your eyebrow awfully put into effect your stage of life. Row lift make the top half of the face look long and elegant or otherwise looking at the sleepy eyebrows whom do you think will attract?

In an attempt to lift your eyebrows, your goal should be to tighten the skin around and trim the mass of skin between the eyebrows and eyelash and fresh faced.

The rest work which I told you for the structures around eyes definately strengthen the muscles around eyebrows and to some extend don't let the eyebrows fall to the lowest point. Along with this one exercise due to which you yourself soon will get some relief from the falling eyebrows, whom I also do this.

Rest your whole palms on your face and put the middle fingers of both the hands underneath each eyebrow. Keep your eyes open and with these middle fingers bring your eyebrows upwards and then outwards. Keep this position for few seconds. Then press your eyebrows against your own fingers, keeping your eyes open. Hold this position for few seconds. Repeat.

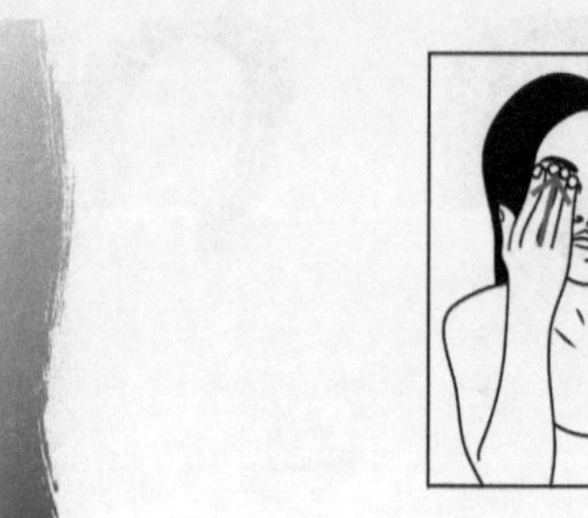 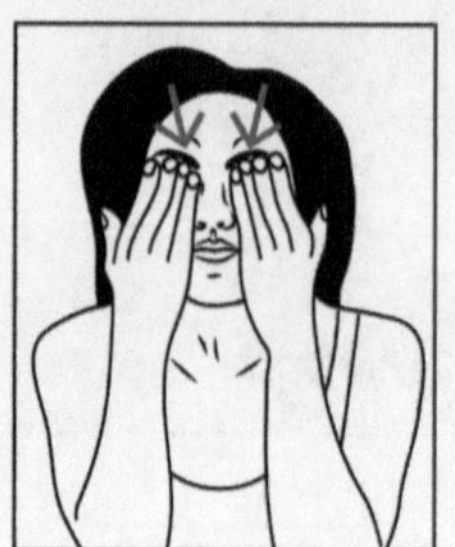

Saggy Eyelids

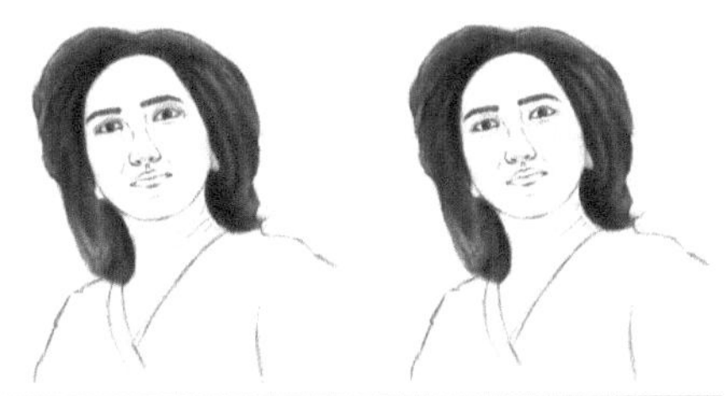

Human body is the greatest work of art explored by ancient Egyptians pharaohs, painters, photographers and bestowed their elements of art by engaging themselves in cave rocks, sculptures and drawings.

In recent years, these medium of communication has also undergone fundamental change. Todays monomania is fashion, which serves as an instant language to enhance the appearance, very well by make-up artists who skilfully transform human canvas creating the perfect illusion, for whom everyone gets obsessed with and imitate.

I waded through a fashion magazine where Chole Savigny during her resort collection opening ceremony was even obsessed with really pink eyelids which the singer of Cocteau twins used to do and following her makeup artist tediously enhancing the appearance of her face, she said "I'm really into a blush on the eyelid and on the high of the cheek" and even she was caught admiring the little romance the really pink eyelids added to the cool outfits.

Think, what if you doesn't get an enough space to paint your eyelids, when it sags?, would your make up, eyeliner, eyeshadow able to see under the excess skin? would you be able to give your desired message of personifying your romance? What would you do to make better of your saggy eyelids and improve your physical appearance, self confidence and make them feel more charming and attractive? Would you go for fillers underneath the sensitive eyes, or use laser procedures to tighten the sink under the eyelid? Is it a must have for living? to get rejuvenated or rested appearance?

What could be done within our reach is that we could add some small inclusions by ourselves so as to sustain the process of aging, somewhat.

You know, the upper eyelid is controlled by the levator palpebral muscle, so we can work on this muscle to prevent droopy eyelids.

To Strengthen Droopy Eyelid

Put your finger under the eyebrow in that position that you could hold the brow bone firmly. Then slowly close your eyes. Pull your eyebrows up with eyelids. Then squeeze the eyelids tightly together to create a stronger pull. Keep that position for 5 seconds. Repeat 5–10 times a day.

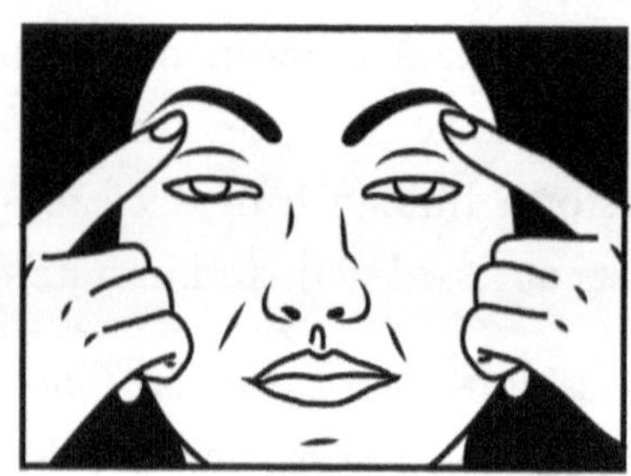

To Strengthen the Tone of Delicate Eye

Sit in a relax place and close your eyes. Now put an index finger on each eyelid

Keep elbows straight outside of the body. Now slowly put some pressure with the pads of your index finger on eyelids. Still applied with pressure, open eyes after 5 seconds. Repeat for 5–10 times.

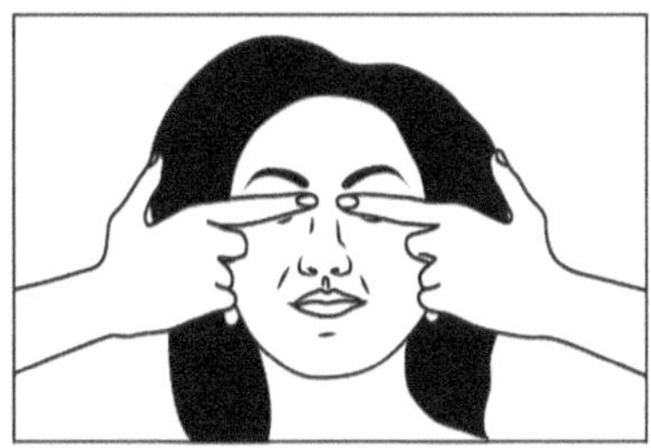

Strengthening the Muscles of the Eyebrow Area

Trying to strengthen to the muscles of the eyebrow area, could help to give a good shape to the saggy eyelids. For that, raise your eyebrows as high as you can put high. Then open your eyes as widely and keep this position for 5 seconds. After, low your eyebrows and be relax. Repeat for some time.

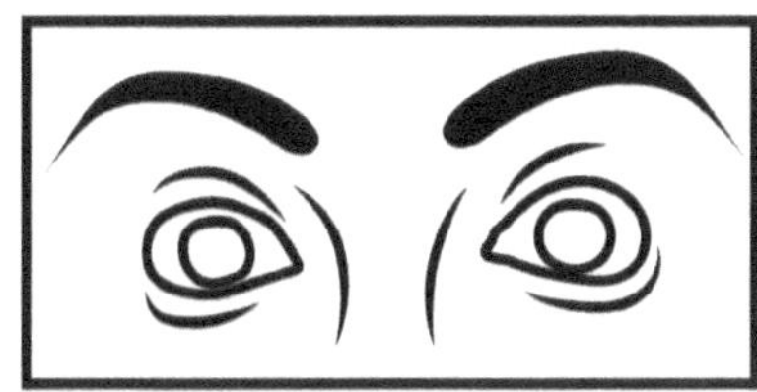

Crows Feet

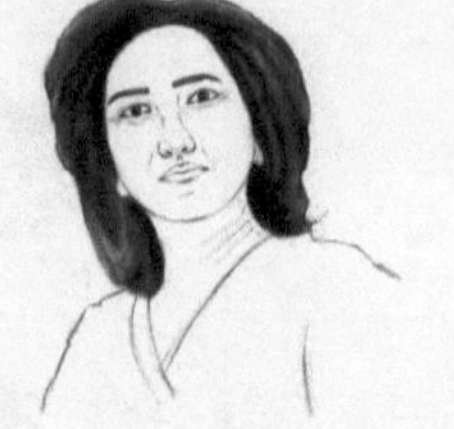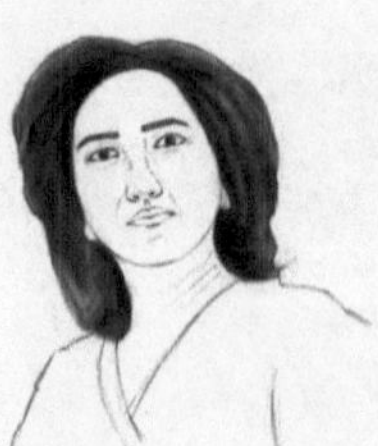

Almost nothing need to be said when we have eyes as an interpreter and the perky wrinkles which radiates from the corner of the eyes. Yes, these are normal and a sign of well lived life. With age these winkles get deepened to bear resemblance to the spitting image of "crows feet", to what end I see seduce me as it is learned that it usually comes from a smiling face and is a hallmark of maturity.

Also don't get anxious to know that besides ourselves there are other beings equally competent. For the same reason when someone brings your feet under direction then make sure to hear them a noted crows story of our childhood, that demonstrated the intelligence of crows to choose the heavy objects rather than hollow that would sink to get their food floating. So, don't fret when these crows feet dwell on at the corner of your eyes for the reason research finds that even with almost walnut-sized brains crows can carefully make up their mind before making a decision or reaching a conclusion and achieve impressive cognitive prowess; a manifestation of higher intelligence and analytical thoughts long considered the sole province of human. But still as quite a few friends of mine like to curtail their appearances, I have too nail down everything for the wanderers.

From many exercises, I found the only exercise effective for crows feet, what I tell you too.

Place your index finger by the outer edge of the eyebrow and middle finger on the cheekbone. Next, spread this area between the outer edge of the eyebrow and the cheekbone slightly. Do not form wrinkles near the eyebrow as you are doing this exercise. This movement is very gentle and subtle. Now do this movement on both sides, flare your elbows out and squint your eyes. Hold for 10 seconds as shown in figure. For optimal result I recommend 3 sets, each of 5 repetitions. Thereafter just tap the area between the outer eyebrow and cheekbone.

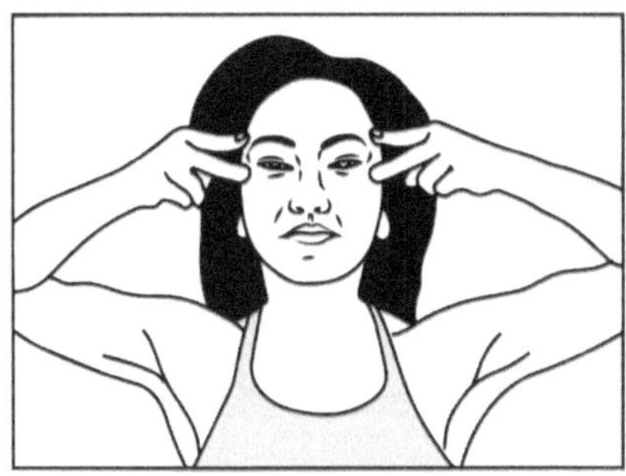

Bags Under Eyes

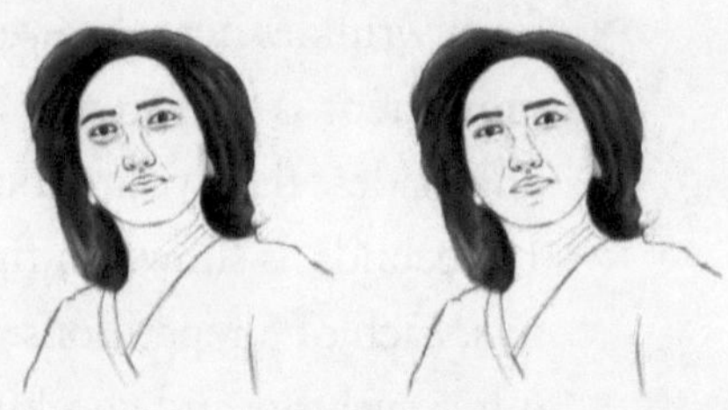

The hills and valleys add to the panoramic scenic beauty but if you find suddenly around and below your eyes, it come off as hag. Those who have creative courage, see these bags differently against the crowd as 'knockoffs', 'Chanel', 'Prada', 'couture' and for some its 'designer eye bags'.

Viewing through the eyes of poets and song writers who put our romantic thoughts and feelings into words by taking help of science, it seems they explain's the bags under the eyes as the body's way of telling us we can carry too much in our hearts. In such a case, being a medical person, I would suggest to make yourself a priority more so than anything else and heed to our predetermined goal.

It is a common complaint and what we often call "bag under the eyes". With aging, the surface facet of the eye changes with muscle lag and gravity, which shifts everything downwards and install on the hills and valleys below the eyes. Depending on whether genetics, thyroid, allergies or aging, the triangular molar moulds appearance varies, also the arch of the bone beneath the eye that forms the prominence of the cheeks varies.

This bag we can find in two context, where changes in the 'fat bag' below eyes comes gradually with aging or inheritance while the 'fluid bag' changes tend to be of shorter duration and it is due to improper nutritional foods, seasonal allergies, insomnia and stress. May occasionally, not often the thyroid or kidney problem cause boggy. Check out your correct reason and work for.

Here all you need is to tone the under eye bags and the well-nigh beneficial exercise I could find is this -

make a "V" sign of your index and middle finger of both hands. Place this V on the outer and the inner corner of the eye. Apply very light pressure to bring your fingers down and try to look up after you get a stretch. Do not wrinkle or frown your forehead. Hold in the squint and close the eyes tightly. Repeat for some time.

Thereafter relax the muscles around eyes by simply revolving the index finger around the eyes.

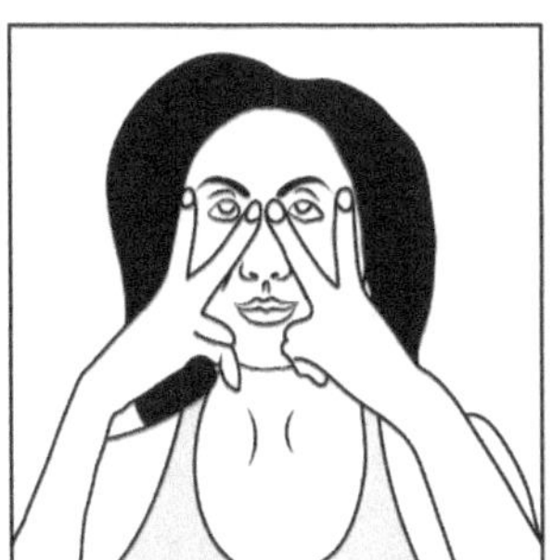 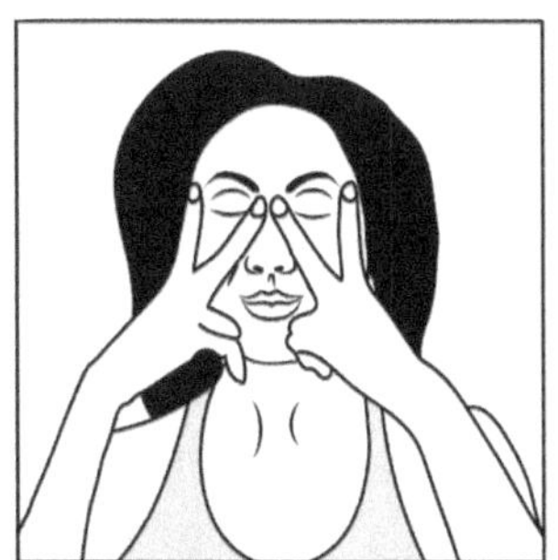

Dark Circles

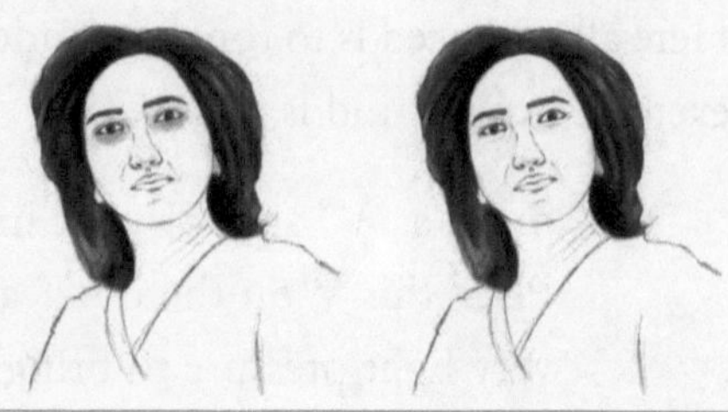

In many instances, when I had to do with dark pigmentation under eyes, I recall my college friend to whom we loved to say "raccoon" for their likeness. Just as raccoon, she was nocturnal, had a relish for junk food and occasionally was rebellious. At the heading edge they both together had an analogy for their dark circles. Those were the pre adulthood times, when falling victim to dark circle speak for heredity while adulthood is when the dark circles are bigger than your friend circle and speaks volumes. About elderly people, humorously many say that they have become so sick of living such a tired life which is quite right, but not as it were anticipated. For me dark circles are not pertaining to tiredness, they are from being awesome, well, its worth getting a few dark circle. Because the causes right from insomnia, stress, aging, certain diseases to the manipulations, misleading done by ecocentric beauty standards by popular culture to the beauty industry playing their mind games all makes the situation horrifying.

My consultation is to scourge away the medical causes and go for optimal.

While writing about for under eye darkness, just a few minutes ago someone asked me if I'm taking yoga workouts? Even though this reference is not expected here, I would like to clarify because this question will be in the minds of more people.

Friends, from any of my conversations, it must to your astonishment that I not ever make use of the term 'yoga' even though existing from India; at which place yogic practices are carried out from earlier times for its distinguished physical and mental effects and aims to use this balanced physical and mental state as an elementary prerequisite to achieve higher state of consciousness, it's because, as matters stood I started resolving them by virtue of the medium of workouts; it was the time of mental instability and uncertainties. Yoga is not just a physical exercise, here we have to make a connect of mind, body and soul to reach the realm of yoga. In those misfortunes(pandemic), where we all were out of fear confined at homes and have had time more than adequate for the needs, my particular challenge was to conduce you, motivate you for workouts, because when everything is falling apart and when very little is in our hands while aging, at rock bottom you should have something on your hands. It's not like that ladies didn't come to me with mental health issues as well, but as those issues comes differently with everyone, needs to be handled individually, a common rationale solution cannot be given. By all means it is for sure, from the medium of workouts, you can in some measures comparatively improve on your state of mind. Definitely trying for concurrent, make my own compendium of the introspected mental issues and bring you to awareness in my next complete composite program in the form of mental therapy.

Although with aging along with your physical likewise your mental health is also of paramount importance. But for certain you will have to be one step ahead in my further work. While taking everyone along, on the name of yoga, I don't want to put a fallacy of the significance of yoga for its unparalleled mind/body modality. I didn't want to misinterpret the advantages of yoga for it comply a different aspect, which otherwise, someone just comes out of a coma and start giving irresponsive claims on the name of yoga. Yoga is self disciplining your body and mind to achieve a 'peaceful' body and mind, from external awareness to internal awareness.

Once you get aware of your physical self from the way of workouts, in my next work, I will latch onto my surge into internal awareness, then further comes the stage of mental health, to obtain that stage I finally will use yoga, which will be explicated from my next work in the form of various asanas.

Every last one of us is a slave of age and we have to play laughingly surrender it, because we can do just little to get free against the law of this incessant nature. Along these lines your dark circles to get visible is eternal with your poor blood circulation and insufficient toxin drainage from the delicate under-eye area. In such dilemma most exact and epistemic, is to increase blood flow to your face and if you have the desire and determination to do, here's a method for accomplishing it.

Stretching the muscles of whole body stand straight and stretch your hands upwards. Start bending slowly until your palms mange to touch the floor and your head touches the knee. Keep breathing deeply. Then stretch your arms forward and up, slowly come to the standing position. Breathing out, bring your arms to the side.

It does not matter how slow you are progressing, as such you won't be able to see the result instant, but think, you are still ahead of everyone who isn't trying.

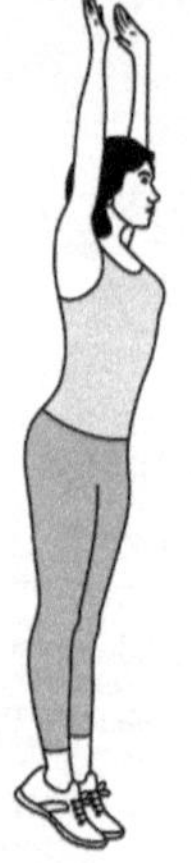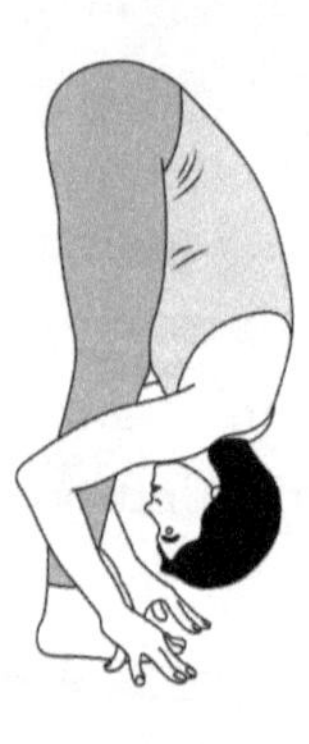

Bed Hangs

To perform this exercise, lie on bed with your legs stretched out and let your head hang over the edge of bed. Now, slowly raise your head and bring the chin to your chest, stay in a position for ten seconds as shown in figure, relax your head and repeat for about five times.

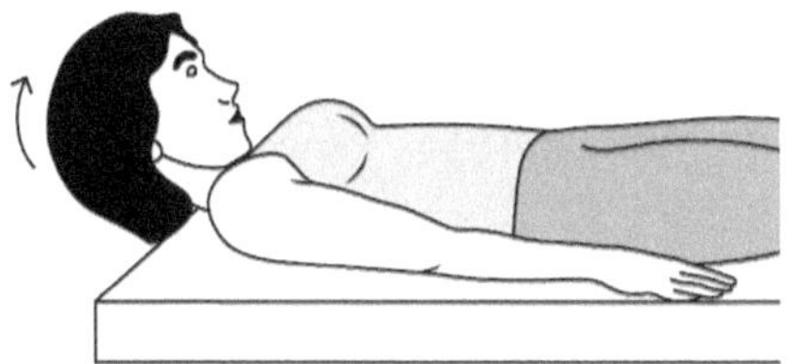

To Relieve Stress Relaxing Your Eye Muscles

Sit down and breath normally. Start looking at the spot between your eyes, for a count of five and then relax. Now, again look at the tip of your nose and count five.

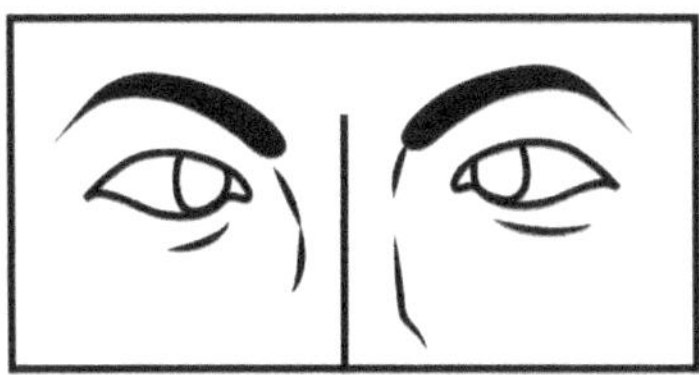 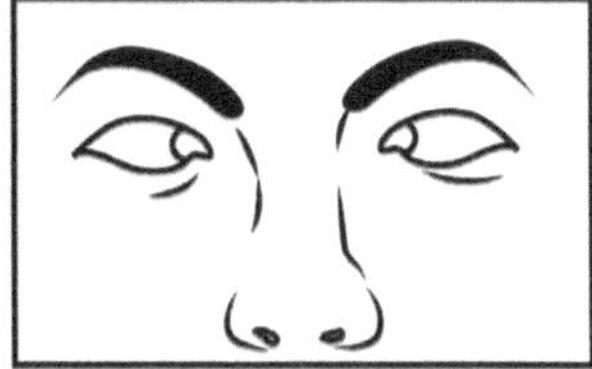

To Lighten the Dark Circles Massage Would Help

Pat the area around the eyes gently with the fingertip of your index finger, without exerting too much pressure and do this smoothly.

Begin to be Oblige to Combat Dehydration

Leading a busy life can sometimes turn even a simple stuff like drinking enough water into a daily challenge. In consequence you might be walking around with a mild case of dehydration without even realising it and could contribute to under eye puffiness. In such case, replenish the fluid level in the body by consuming clear fluids such as water, clear broths to flush out the toxins from your system and thereby reducing the amount of salt concentration in

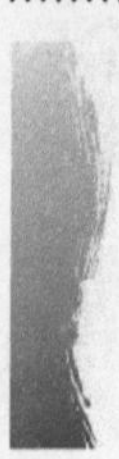

and around the eyes. And if you are daily exercising make sure you are receiving enough fluids.

Apart from exercise, apply ice cubes to refresh eye area and thereafter aloe gel with vitamin E oil under your eyes every night.

Nose Drooping

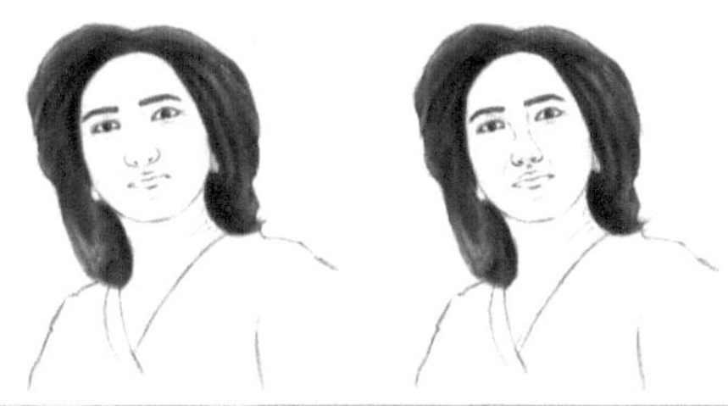

Nose is esteemed as leading facial profile and part of well known academic exercise where the character sketch of nose is usually identified as perceived truth using tools like irony, humour, exaggeration and satire. Usually identified in a manner when a woman want to visit lavatory, she excuses by saying "I will be right back, just have to powder my nose".

Often women are spotted to have a nose for bargain. It is no secret of her to intrude into others affair or even that really doesn't concern her, still she wants to stick her nose into. As far as to draw readers in, "right under one's nose", "keep your nose clean" and some more idioms are used to amplify messages and helps to awaken their senses. Similarly considering facial features, when the tip of nose droop, it underscores to sizeable impact on all in all illusion of face.

This ptosis come about when the tip of the nose is more caudal than what is deemed idle. With age, the tip-supportive mechanism and de-rotation of the nasal tip weakens by dismissing the continuity of the lateral and medial crura of the lower cartilage of nose. Also the cartilage with which it is sculptured break off as we age and happen to droop nose and look bigger.

The oversize nose for a persons face is well conceded when the nose is longer than 2.2 inches for a man or 2 inches for a woman. Further for getting aesthetically perfect nose, you may aspire to loose nose fat, also to earn composite teeny-weeny nose, sharpened nose, short nose or slim-jim nose.

Like you asked me many a time herein a couple of workouts to sculpt the desirable nose sooner or later.

Nose Sagging

Friends, we have often heard of the house sags its flooring or the damaged stills and joint ends that contribute to them, often involves jacking. Here the common scenario is to install temporary jack posts and support beams, a taut string stretched across the floor shows improvement in its deflection. Here you could see the aim is not for perfection, but simply stability and improvement. After all, if perfectly level floor were important to us, we wouldn't live in old houses, would we?

Similarly, what we should expect for the sagging nose other than only a taut stretch? after all. If perfectly levelled nose were important to us like the perfectly level floor, we wouldn't live in old houses, would we? Why would we live in old houses then? Only here I turned out the excerpt of aging under the pretext of construction facts.

That's all you have to do, jack some pressure with your index fingers at the side of your nose and breath out with force, but not too much. Apply pressure on the bottom of the nostrils, if you can. Repeat for 10 times.

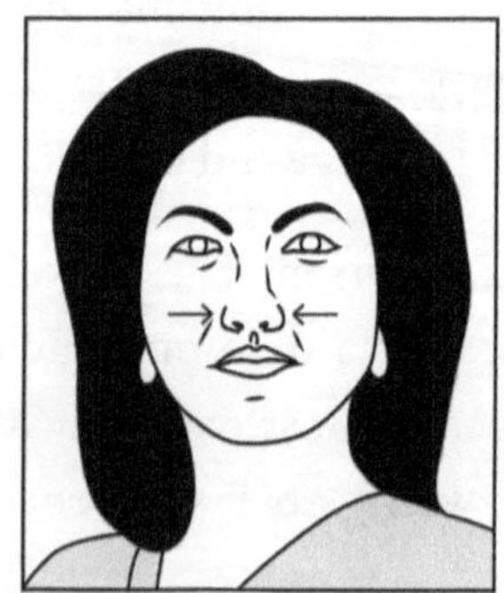

To Reshape the Nose and Firm the Muscles Around the Nose Area

Hold your nose with index and thumb of one hand and press the tip of the nose towards the face in upward direction with the index finger of other hands shown in figure. Now bring the upper lip down and count 1,2 and bring back the upper lips, do it 5–10 times for 3 sets.

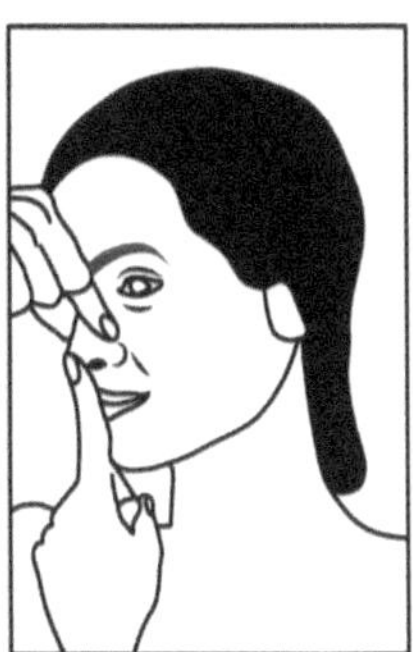

To Sharpen Your Nose

Make a smile and push the tip of your nose upwards with the index finger for few times a day.

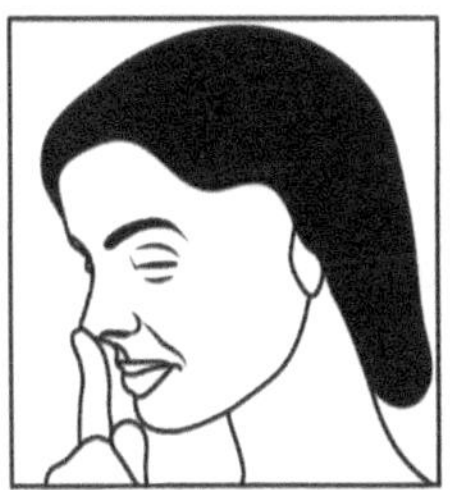

To Shorten Your Nose

This simple exercise besides shaping your nose, shortening your nose, but will also prevent deterioration of your nose cartilage.

Place your index finger on the tip of your nose and push it gently as shown in figure. Now, serve your nose to exert downward pressure on the finger as shown in figure so as many times a day.

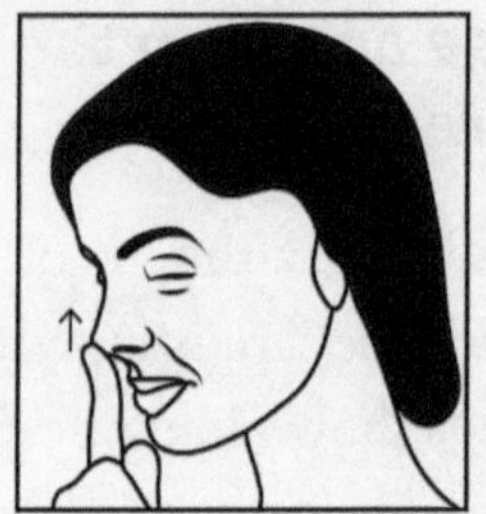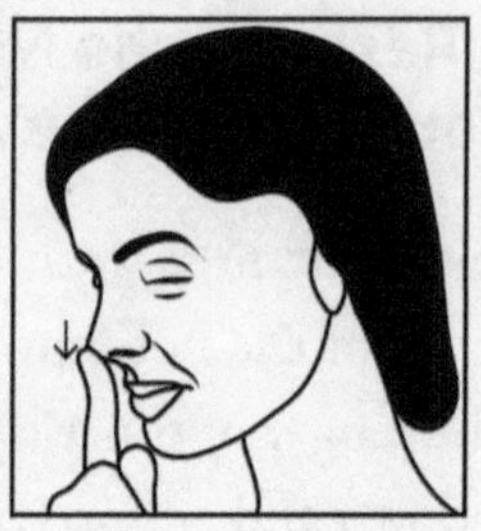

Alternately pinch your right nose and breath air in from left nostril other similarly pinch your left nostril and exhale air out from the right nostril. Similarly, next repeat with starting by your left nostril. Do for at-least 10 times.

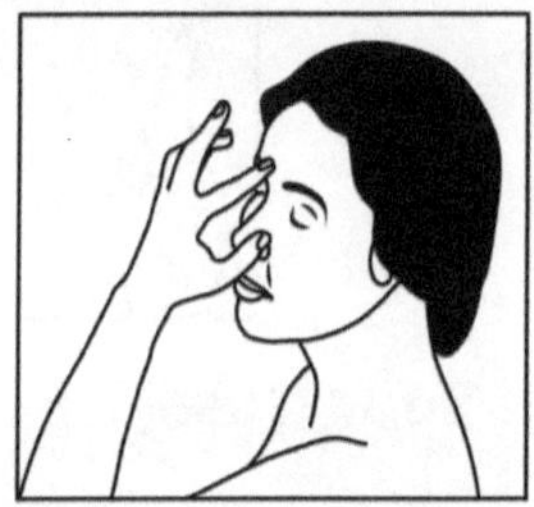

To Strengthen Nose - "Wiggle"

If you had been the science student, you would had definitely noticed the "wiggle" of earthworm during your practicals of zoology in the laboratory. For its wiggle, earthworm uses its powerful and well developed circular and longitudinal muscles to work together which helps them to push its way through the substratum of the soil. Similar, in humans, for strengthening the nasal muscles, "wiggle" is done with the help of 'nasalis' muscle of the nose which functions to compress the nasal cartilage and responsible for flaring of the nostrils and 'depressor septic muscle' responsible for drawing the nose downward.

For wiggling, you don't need to move your face, keep it still overall. Only move your nostrils up and down. It should feel like you are pulling your nose down towards your mouth and when you relax your face, your nose should go back to into place. Do it vigorously for some time.

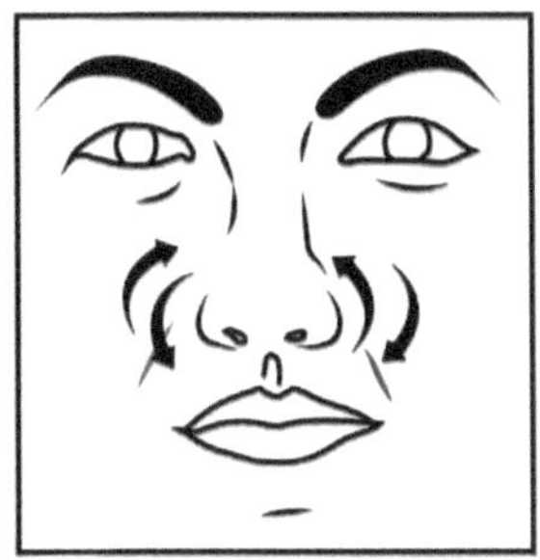

To Narrow Your Nose - "Massage"

Using two fingers of your two hands start from the top of nose and go down to the bridge and down to the sides. Do this with clockwise motion on one hand and counter clockwise motion on the other.

Perplexity of Cheeks

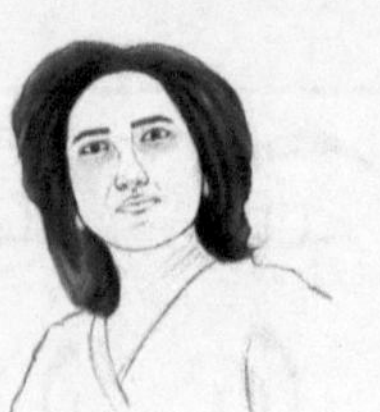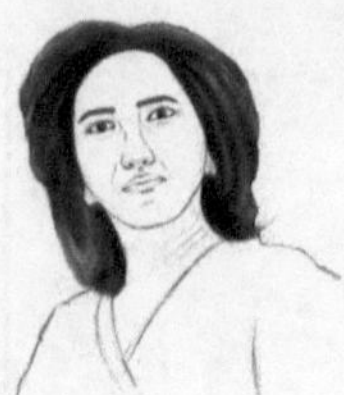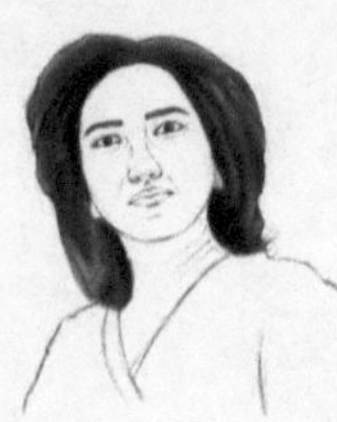

Time changes everything. Over the years I realise that a year can do a lot to a person, it could make you grow and understand things, also at the same time it do not let you forget the old you. Then why understanding of our coveted physical traits not even?

I will reminisce those gone days, how his kiss made my cheeks pink, how did he get mesmerised by my baby cheeks, how my cheeks responded to the cold winter nights by getting pink and now how with fall of oestrogen the hot flushes is forging my cheeks pink.

My mother was unenlightened of all these ever. For them, fuller cheeks is a sign of well fed home and that was looking obvious. Today also I get touched by her chubby cheeks. There is definately some change in them with age but while laughing still these mounds are seen there. A question comes that will my daughter's approach on this consideration match us? Today's girls want them to do scissor on everything what is excess. How could she like chubby cheeks? You may be inclined to think some other interesting physical traits of your family, search a little.

This is the only subject, to know it, when I pushed myself to know the precise meaning of what they said, I got thrown off balance but gathered my willingness and finally set the seal on them.

Some women's chubby cheeks gift them youthful appearance; and if they cling intact till late, then it's a matter of honour, whereas, somes chubby cheeks give their face a bloated appearance to whom they make up by sucking cheeks and pushing out the lips to contorts the face in congruence with touchstone of cover girl. Contrary elsewhere, the sunken hollow cheeks manifests wrinkles and ill health. Then somewhere else, as it seem exotic and draws attention with any of hair length, high cheek bones fascinates women. Looking at the growing trend of social media, in want of 'perfect selfie', to frame a perfect angle wants higher cheeks bones while some die for voluptuous cheeks to enhance more beauty in photos and selfies.

It is your requisite, but certain medical conditions also alter your cheeks appearance and make them swell like some allergies, sinusitis, thyroid, fluid retention, Cushing syndrome, angioedema, actinomycosis, cancers, certain medication. Sunken cheeks (which often expose your cheek bones) is although a sign of natural aging could be due to loss of subcutaneous fat, eating disorders like bulimia, anorexia, tuberculosis, dehydration, tobacco smoking, extreme exercise, also from not getting enough sleep, extreme weathers.

What I anticipate from you? lay bare the situation well to your doctors and do what needs to be done.

It's quite interesting to know that the order in which our body stores fat in the opposite order it reduces the fat. like the order of fat gain is abdomen, hips, thighs, buttocks, face, and while reducing face comes first. When the process of weight loss started in me, rather than my body, my face conquer the attention of my friends first. But seeing my cheeks she understood me as sick.

My contemplative nature started thinking whereas my workouts are not ending the aesthetic of my face. Exclusively the aforesaid reason caught my attention and I understood my workout plan is working. And nevertheless if possible I had to exercise every single muscle of the body which I used to do. In the immediate future, the way my muscles, by conjoining with the frame of the face shaped them, I was astonished to see the contours of my face. Now, my cheeks sound enough elegant like they should have been according to my facial skeleton. So, do not be doubtful even a little. While performing the rest of physical activities you can equally try to lift cheeks or slim them.

Kiss-Kiss Fish

Whenever I get a chance to speak about cheeks, I doesn't forget to memorize how Mr. Fish all of a sudden turned into a Kiss-Kiss Fish from a Pout-Pout Fish after he is kissed by shimmering silver fish. Came to see when a kiss is put to test, it transformed Mr. Fish life into happiness and purpose in life. Just like that many activities seem like a waste but if it gives you happiness than why not? Similarly, if by making an exaggerated kissing face with your two lips would make you happy as it gives your visage slimmer stronger appearance, then why not? Purking up and sticking your lips out with regards and making a smooching sound you yourself push out and release bringing your lips back to rest, can be enjoying along with solving your purpose for slender cheeks. Repeat this move for 10–20 times.

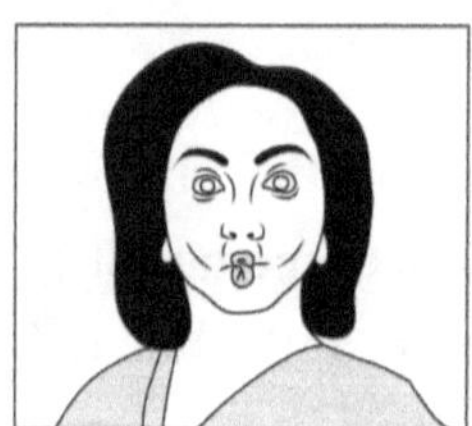

Oh Sexy

It doesn't matter what age you are, I think, if you look sexy, feel great and say "Oh sexy" to yourself few times during the day, I bet who would not admire you. The way your face muscles moves while saying these gives your face a well toned and slimmer appearance.

Propel Your Tongue

There are certain rare talents you probably don't have like raising your single eyebrow, wiggling of ears, sneezing with your open eyes and touching your tongue to nose. Do not panic, this talent appear among 10 % people. Even so we all can defiantly take our tongue over the upper lips. That's what needed for our next workout. Open your mouth and try to reach your tongue to the upper margin of your upper lips. looking down you will see your mounted cheeks. Hold this position for some time. If further along with chubby cheeks you want to strengthen your jaw then point your chin towards the ceiling while doing this move as shown in figure.

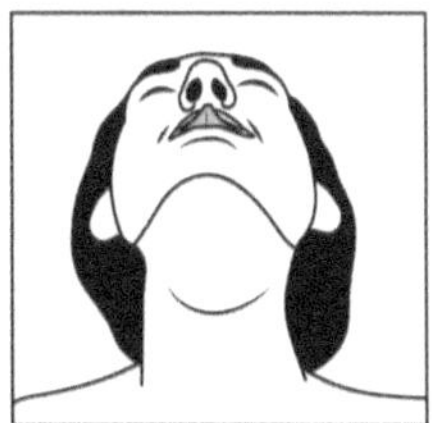

Puppet Face Move

No one can fail to remember how the puppets looks like. They show off their teeth with mouth wide open and a deep crease is crafted from the mouth deep towards chin so puppeteers can help them talk. Partake in this activity by smiling wide and pressing your fingertips into the creases between the nose and lips. Now uplifting the cheek (as shown in figure) circulate your fingertips in circular motion to prevent it from becoming saggy.

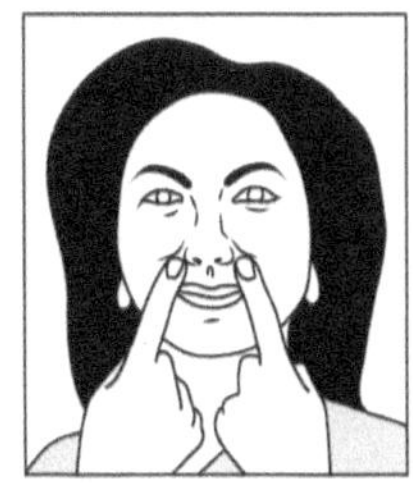

Depuff Your Face

Among the other possibilities your impaired lymphatic circulation could be one of the cause of face swelling and puffiness, in which the toxins and metabolic wastes gets accumulated in the cells below your skin

In such case massage your face with gentle circles of your fingers. Start at the top of the face, then around your eyes and then slowly below cheeks then towards your jaws.

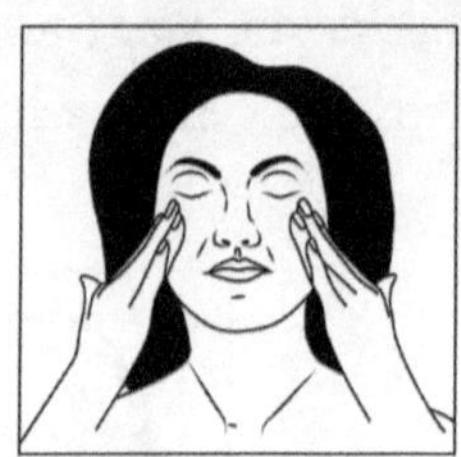

In a postscript I want to make you aware of the nasty complications of filler injections causing black rotting flesh hard, lumpy lips and nasty bacterial infections which can lead women permanently disfigured. In a defence to brag their superiority they ask whether the claims of face workouts are actually well-founded and worth your time? Despite all the stories, without getting into controversies, I want every single muscle of my body oxygenated (the benefits of which are obvious), for whom I keep trying.

Nasolabial Folds

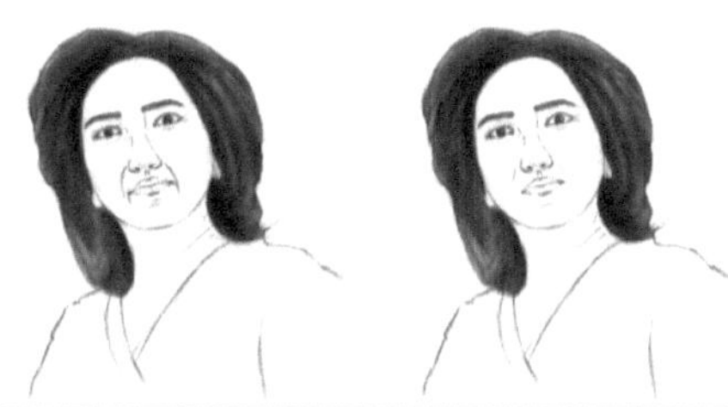

Mouth area is the sole solitary site on your face that could perhaps may well develop wrinkles; who is a greeting sign of aging. For me, it's the harvest of old age one reap in the form of laugh lines and that result from the collection and abundance of blessings previously secured. So, its the right time to embrace your aging gracefully in its existing form, constituted by nature.

But with age, in some, these lines get worst when they get deeper and longer and can even reach jawline. When problem free is the way to be and when there is time in hand; there is nothing bad in minimising them.

Wrinkles that built around the mouth happen to come in the nature of -

'Smile lines' which are formed from the bottom corners of nose towards far and wide of your mouth, 'marionette lines' pleat around the mouth and declines the corner of your mouth, while other worrying factors which escalate years to an otherwise youthful complexion are 'lip wrinkles' or 'lipstick lines' that are vertical just above your upper lip and are badly difficult to hide. This loss of tone and succeeding collapse of skin on the upper lip is not due to elongation as with most facial muscle but rather due to lack of circulation that the lips looses its outline, becomes thinner and brindles. Here, all you could visualise is the aging effect, but don't let it get you down and if you let, it's too hard to get back up. Act on time.

The Mouthwash Move

All you need to do is fill your mouth with air instead of mouthwash and swish the air in all directions as you would do with mouthwash, while holding for about five seconds in each area. Once each area is touched upon, release the air. Repeat few more times.

if you see your lips are getting dry, cracking, flaking and peeling, you can fill your mouth with one teaspoon of coconut oil added to some water and swish it all directions or can just hold it for few minutes inside mouth. This will combat any inside inflammation and act as an emollient which helps to soothe and soften your lips.

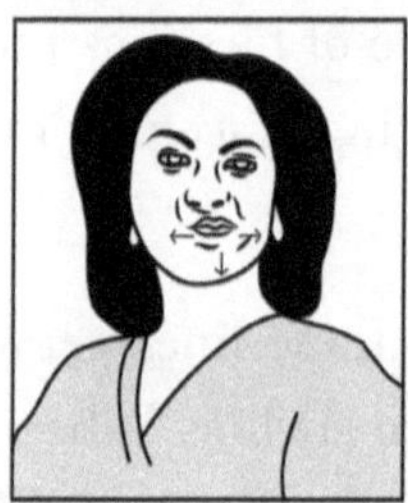

Lip Press

It not only builds the orbicularis oculi muscles that surrounds the whole mouth, also add fullness to the lips and the surrounding area. Wrap your lips over your teeth and masticate down as would be the case of swelling. Apply enough pressure between the teeth, work from right to left then left to right until you feel strained or enough for one minute.

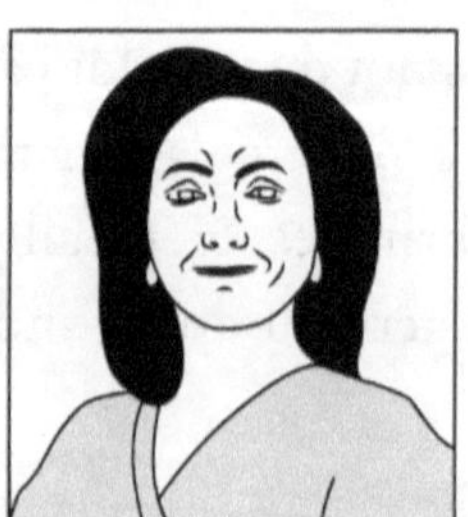

Squeeze

If you want to get rid of the vertical lines above lips enhance the circulation around it by gently squeezing the lips together from right to left and left to right.

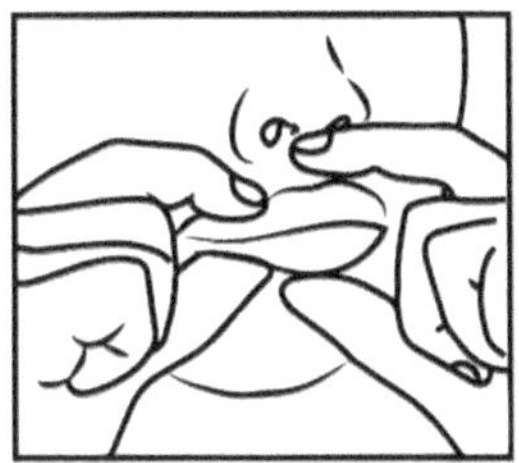

Sagging Jowls

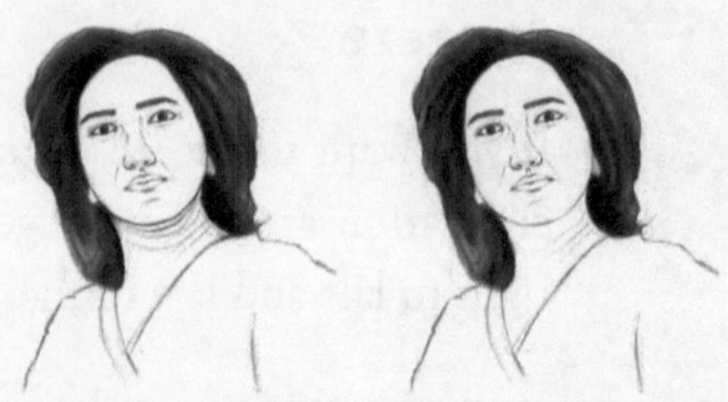

Before all else mankind catch sight of your face, its little wonder that we are often absorbed in wishing for ravishing looks. Also you and I assess people on the blink of their demeanour. Whereas, depending upon the male and female facial distinguishing peculiarity, our forefather used to forecast the health and fertility of your spouse.

Often in gym, your trainer creates a tailored fitness and wellness plan for individuals and groups, also teach popular conditioning methods such as pilates for yoga, planks for posture, dips for chest and squats for muscles of thighs, hips and buttocks. Means they have across from further the many workouts for hundreds of muscles extensively, but why not for face? which also consists of a group of about 20 flat skeletal muscles which are wholly unattended in gym workouts. Presuming your body can bestow your desired convert after workouts, remarkably your face muscles can, although there is little evidence of face exercises. Think, unlike micro needling or a chemical peel a workout can't hurt, rather might help.

If truth be told on a deep psychological level about men, chiselled body with plump face is a great no-no for me. But allowing both, chisellers body and defined jawline is heart stopping. Alone defined jawline would say is a buzzer to women's brain reasoning the rest of the body is chiselled too.

Don't you want to see yourself attractive by making the noticeable distinction between the jaw and the neck by clinging out the mandible bone? irrespective of your neckline. Look, how would it look like pairing necklaces with neckline that too with chiselled jawline? Wouldn't it flaunt your sense of proficiency in aesthetics?

As the extra fat in the neck and jaw area come into sight or embark to shrink with age, the jawline becomes less defined. With length of time, you can't exchange blows with aging and genetics but you can make better your jawline. See, your aesthetics and aging go hand in hand. So, when we work both ways at the same moment in unison with each other, I think, it would be nice if you could have the jewel in the crown.

While talking about for neck, when you see yourself in front of the mirror, precisely what do you see? and what do you feel when you touch this region? Yes, you see the "turkey neck" and while touching you palpate the wax and wane of plexus, blood vessels, lymphatics and muscles and feel the pulsations over. So, viewing the complexity of structure there, one should be thoughtful and cautious in ones action. Here, for the objective to achieve, we have to target the muscles attach from sternum and collar bone to various parts of the jawbone.

After compiling and assessing the evidence, we can conclude that neck exercises produce visible aesthetic results. If you want to increase your face value and burn Rome to ground, I bet, decent face, elegant chiseled jawline and a smile would work wonders. With why not to work right under the nose for your heartfelt facial expression - "smile".

Neck Curl Up

This entice the front neck muscles. As the neck muscles are underdeveloped, doing in haste could bring strain on your neck muscles, so hold your horses.

Lie on your back with the tongue pressed on the roof of the mouth. Bring your chin to your chest and then lift your head off the ground about 2 inches keeping rest of the body at rest.

Initially start for 10 repetitions of 1 set and you can gradually move to more.

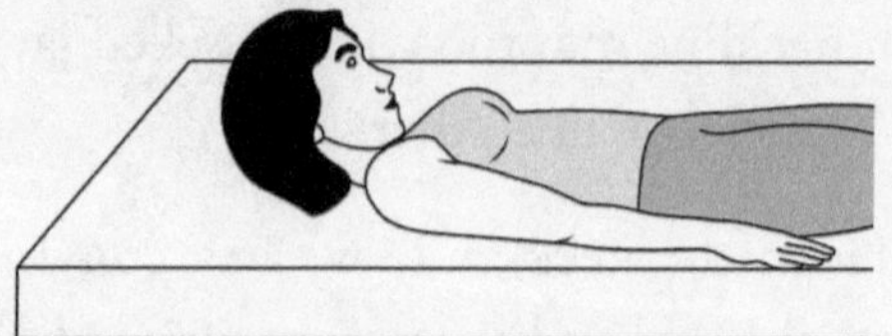

Tongue Twister

To target the muscles underneath the chin, place your tongue onto roof of your mouth directly behind your teeth and press your tongue to completely close the roof of your mouth and add tension. Then begin humming and making a liberating sound, this will activate the muscles.

Vowel Sounds

For working the muscles around mouth and the side of your lips, start with your mouth open and say "A", "I", "E", "O", one after another, exaggerate the sound and try not to touch or show your teeth.

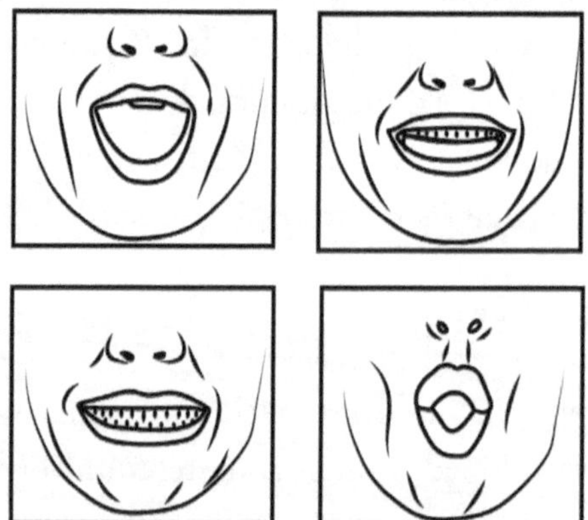

Chin Up

lift the face and chin muscles with your mouth closed, push your lower jaw out and lift your lower lip. Feel the stretch build just under the chin and in the jawline. Hold for 10–15 seconds, then relax. Initially perform 1 set of 10 repetitions thereafter increase sets.Or you can simply stretch your jaw out and feel the stretch.

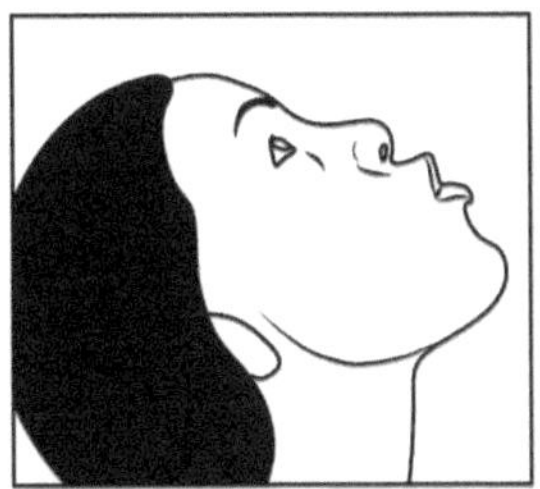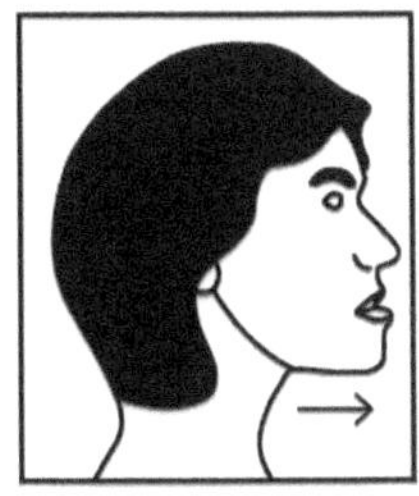

Sagging Chin Exercise

Place your elbow on a table with your fist under your chin, then try to open your mouth while exerting force with your rest to create resistance. Hold than release.

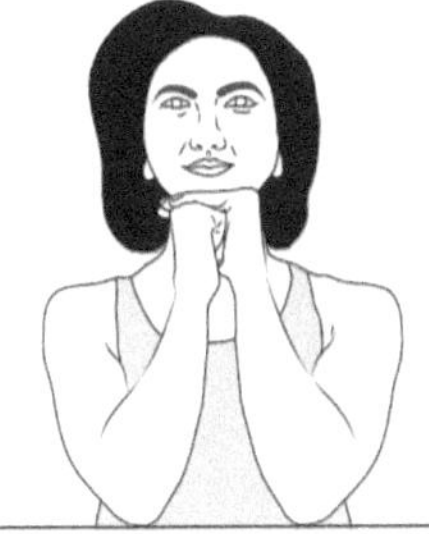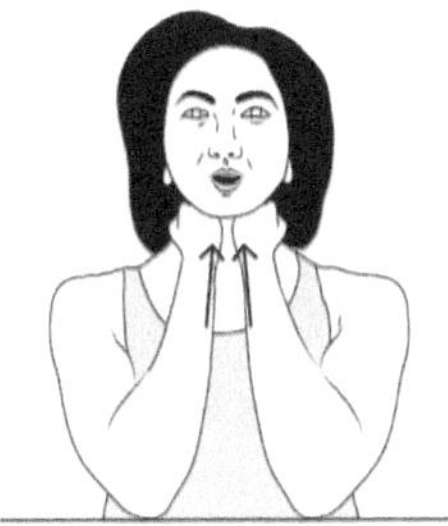

Jaw Bone Restore

Put your thumb below your chin, side by side. Then slightly push your chin down, creating resistance, and slowly slide your thumbs along your jawline to your ears.

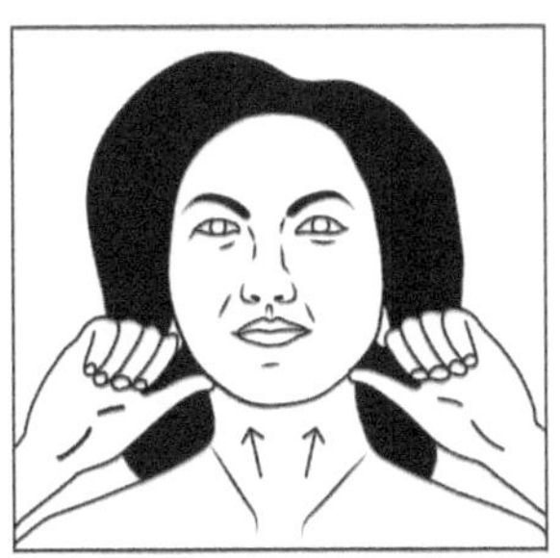

Jawzrsize facial toner

Jawzrsize face exerciser is a ball, which comes in various resistance and its been said that it strengthens over 50 muscles in your face and neck but I never made its use. For you I insist to carry it only after counselling your doctor before.

Hunch Back

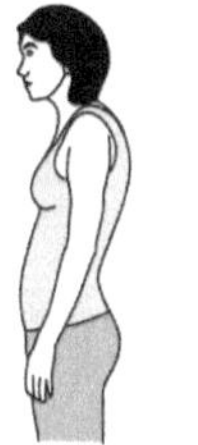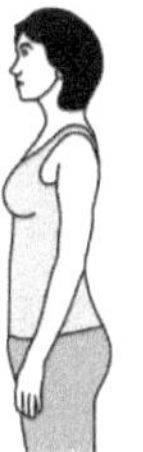

Out of the preconceived notions, I went through aversion towards flipping along my photograph album memories until one day I came across on my table an album of the medical seminar held in recent past at my college, thereupon changed my psyche to "every photo is a mirror image of ourselves and has much more story to tell".

I am in no way contrary to human nature having a natural drive of admiring exclusively owns photographs. And suddenly my eye caught hold of the one, where although I was well favoured, my hunched shoulder and forward head disappointed me. Looking back, recollecting the memories of seminar, I discovered my digging head for long working hours over months and the muscle knots between the shoulder blades, the upper back and in the lower leg were been among the major reasons for my bad posture that time. Soon I gained the understanding of proper posture and incorporated uniform mixture of- to stand tall, sit correct, to move around at least a few minutes every hour, wall slides, child pose, shoulder blade squeeze with plank and bridges, and within a short span I corrected my mechanical back pain and posture that stick around into my lifestyle.

Till now I knew that, this stage comes when, in that phase of life when for a long time our spoiled posture, gravity and bone strength decreases. But, today it's also in the hit-list of youngsters where the present time lifestyle has made them the devotees of smartphone, tablets or laptops and in whose devotion they have become so much indulged that they have forgotten rest worldliness, towards our body.

While working in chair, if you have stiffness in the neck for a little, then it automatically makes hunch back. And if while sitting and you do stretching correctly, so you can bring a lot of change. If you often forget things then program your apparatus to remind you for stretching and to get up and take a walk around. For stretching, while seated just pull your shoulders back and squeeze your shoulders blades together also tuck in your chin in forward and then backward feeling the stretch.

If you experience neck pain, back pain, so because of muscles, ligaments and joints, but frequent hip and back pain include injury to muscles from overuse, disc injury ,degeneration due to age or spinal stenosis resulting in tenderness over the facet joints, decreased movements and stiffness, pain in bending backwards and pain in buttocks or radiating pain down the thigh(sciatica). These troubles should be immediately rectified by doctors initially, next with their advice exercises like low intensity cardio and weight training activity even can gradual unequivocally bring together.

Upper back area of the body includes the shoulder blades and where the rib cage connects to the chest region and often experienced as pain or discomfort throughout the back side of the chest. In these conditions following exercises gives a great relief-

A Doorway Stretch (Pectoral Stretch)

Begin with your facing forward and placing your arms in 90-degree position at the door frame. Next, slowly lean forward until you feel a slight stretch in your shoulders. Hold the stretch for few breaths and relax. Repeat.

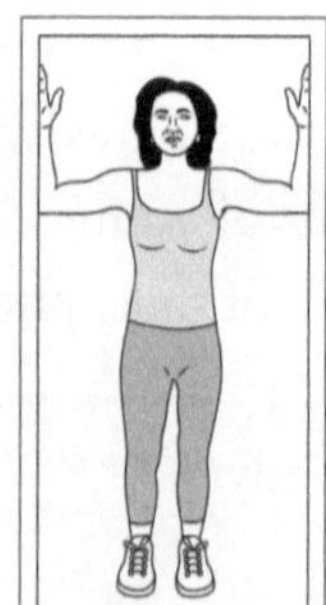

Upper Trap Stretch

An upper trap can be done seated at your desk. Sit up tall and look forward. Next, slowly without lifting your shoulders and tilting your head try to bring your ear to your shoulder. More stretch can be felt by using your hand to give slight extra pressure. Start with 2–3 times and hold for 20–30 seconds at a time.

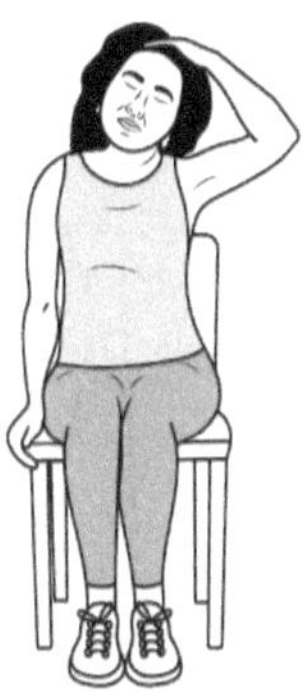

Strengthening Your Upper Back

Some strengthening exercises to start with are scapular squeezes, prone I and prone T's.

Scapular Squeeze

A scapular squeeze is performed sitting (or standing) with your elbows bent and palms forward. Thereafter bring about your shoulders back and slightly downwards, squeezing your shoulder blades together. Start with a five-second squeeze and try to complete 10. Return to initial position. Repeat.

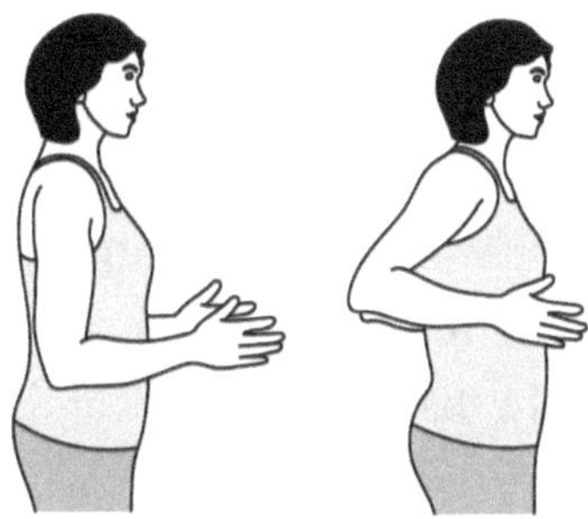

Prone I and T's

Prone I and T's are performed face down on a table (bed or floor can also be used). Roll up a towel and put it under your forehead, arms down at your side (form a letter "I") with palms facing the ceiling, and start to squeeze your shoulder blades together and lift your arms off the table. Do a five-second hold and then lower them back down for 10 time.

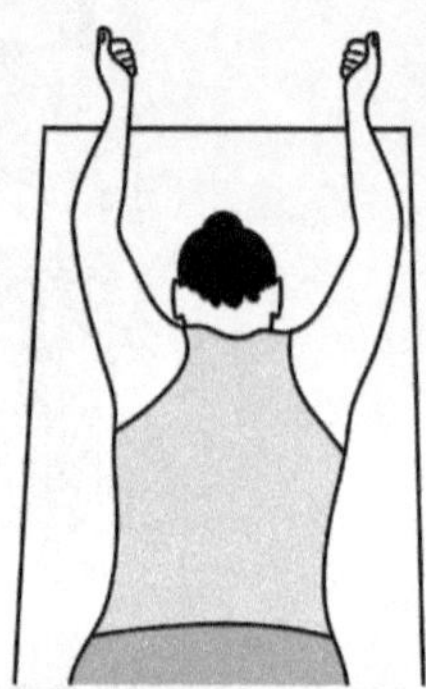

Prone T's are performed in the same position but arms are now moved out to the side . Make fists with your hands then stick out your thumbs and point them towards ceiling. Now squeeze your shoulder blades together and lift your arms up. Do this with a five-second hold for 10 times.

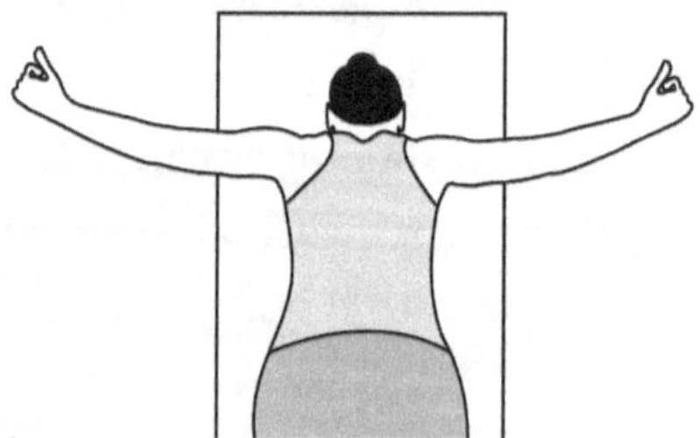

Weight training for bad back

Before strength and weight training with lower back pain, I suggest to take advice from your doctors first. Its critical to strengthen all muscle groups that support back and core, but you can strengthen your shoulders, chest, legs and glutes. Over time, the strength you build in these major areas will help alleviate pressure from the spine, preventing long-term injury. Further to weight train your bad back you can include squats, lunges, push-ups from knees.

Stretches

For the bad lower back you can go for hamstring, quads, glutes stretch to lift pressure from your back. Hamstring stretch can be done by supporting against the wall or gripping towel around the toes. Also go for back press- ups from the floor in push ups position, by keeping your hands planted and lift your upper body off the floor. Hold the stretches for few seconds.

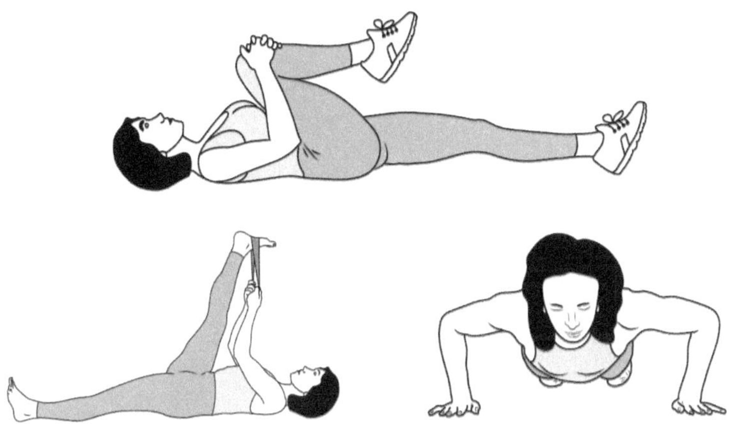

Cardio Activity

Include low impact cardio activity like fast-paced walking for weight loss and to reduce chronic back pain. In gym you can go for using elliptical or step machines.

Aquatic Exercises

Aquatic exercises if you could, equally are useful for the sufferers of back pain.

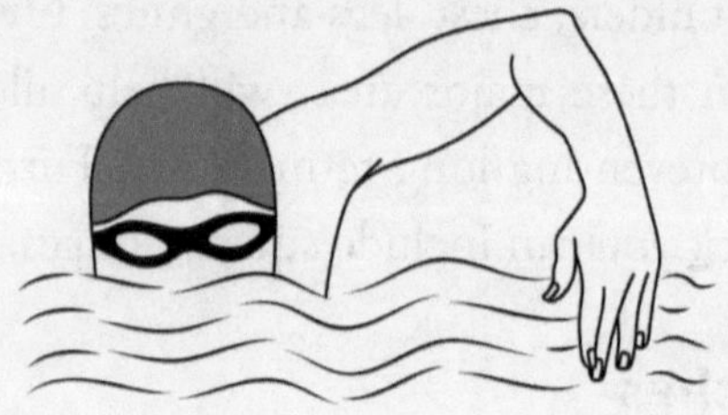

For trigger points you can pressure on the knot for 5–10 seconds and then release it or apply moist hot packs, ice packs to get muscles relax and to decrease pain.

Bat Wings

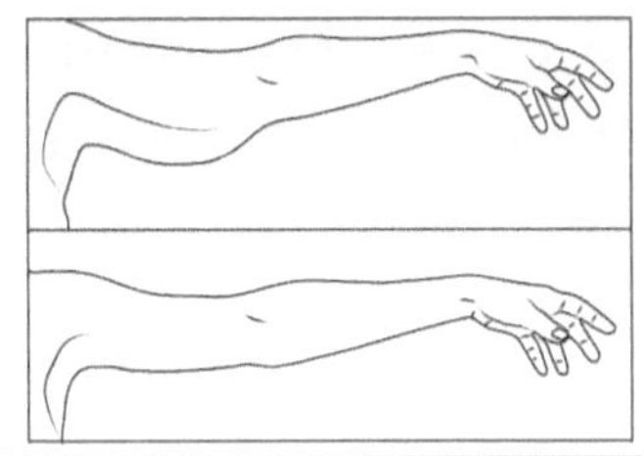

Do you know what it seem to be something when you heard somebody calling your name in the crowd? and you turn to glimpse the smiling faces and waving hands, and know it was for nobody other than you. After I was called for the guest lecture at a health seminar, I was walking on the air when my name was called for felicitation. It was for that moment I first time threw my hands up in the air for receiving everything God is doing in my life and awkwardly waved my hands to react the crowd who of those praised my presentation. More than that, it seemed, my underarm skin enjoyed gracefully to the crowd, seeing that it didn't stop even after I stopped. And why not? It was the exceptional occasion which my arms made the best of to interact with the world, otherwise, arms usually come in ones life for some good byes.

On this drift my son exactly code the different reason. He said that my arms were not waving but were grieving after I neglected them in the process of concentrating in the soft table job apart from my workouts. Probably that could be one of the reason I would had gathered the unwanted attention.

Pertaining to upper body, I was scared for being quite pitiful. Started thinking that to get short lived pleasures, which will give us a simple life we are going to ignore them. I immediately came into action to combat my flabby arms.

While going through the anatomy and physiological aspect of forearm, it's a matter of surprise, humans and bats evolved from the common ancestors. Their forearms, even though look very different externally and deport different functions, include similar bones like humerus, ulna, radius, carpels, metacarpals, phalanges and when the main muscles of the human arms loose their tone, it wobble along with fat to look like bats wings. That's why naming them bats wings may have taken place. In view of the fact, I had to take back my lost muscle tone of upper arm.

Among the two muscles of the upper arm, triceps and biceps, in all intents and purpose, body doesn't use directly tricep muscle, apparently tricep muscle itself wish to sit idle as someone falls in love. However, it's significant to wake up the triceps.

Chasing down the fitness, its desirable to focus on remote areas however it's feasible when you evolve all your body muscle groups. In regards to weight gain, everyone is familiar with the fat prone areas of the thighs, abdomen and arms. If not for calorie burning, at-least to fulfill the wish for wearing the tank top, on what you should act upon?, loose your weight and build your muscles.

Triceps Pushups

We all are well versed with pushups and its confirmed benefits to the entire group of pectorals major muscle group, on the other hand triceps pushups precisely lay emphasis on your upper arms muscles. Also it is found that triangle pushup bring about more action in all three triceps muscles than tricep dips

While regular pushups -with hands slightly farther out and elbows pointed perpendicular to the body, tricep pushups are almost similar to pushups only thing is that while in plank position, with your hands directly under your chest, turn your hands inwards so your fingers form a triangle, which are most appropriate to target the triceps.

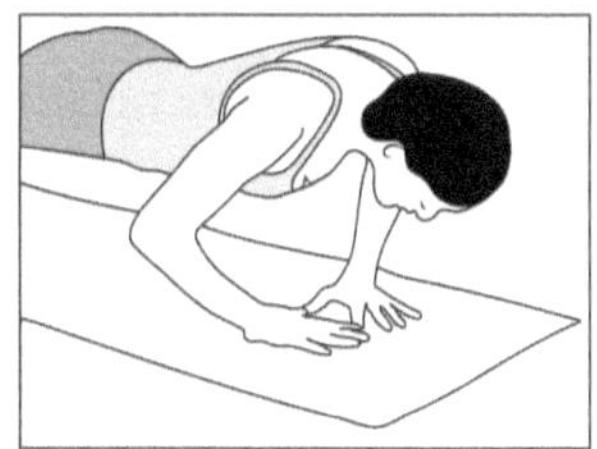

Overhead tricep extension

Start standing with your feet shoulder-width apart. You can either use a single dumbbell or you can work on each arm separately by using two dumbbells in both hands. Keeping your biceps close to your ears and pointing your elbows forward, now raise your dumbbell above your head until your arms are stretched out straight. Slowly lower the weights back behind your head as shown in figure. Do not flare your elbows out too much. Equally keep your biceps close to your ears and elbows pointing forward as you lower the weight behind your head until the elbows are at about 90 degrees angle. Straighten the arms contracting the triceps and then repeat for 1–3 sets of 8–12 reps.

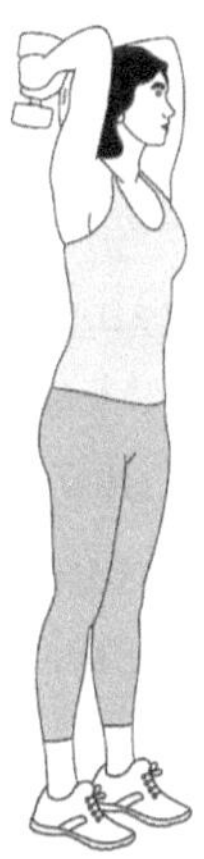

Tricep kickback

Here two positions are crucial. One- your standing position and second- your initial dumbbell position.

At the beginning hold dumbbells in both hands and stand with your legs somewhat apart, knees bent and lean forward slightly(get the exact position as in figure). Now press and hold that dumbbell holding arm against your side, with a 90degree bent at the elbow. Then slowly straighten your one arm backward until it is parallel to the floor. Take a short pause. Slowly lower your arm back at 90degree angle. Repeat for 12–15 repetitions. Similarly do with another arm. Try 2–3 sets.

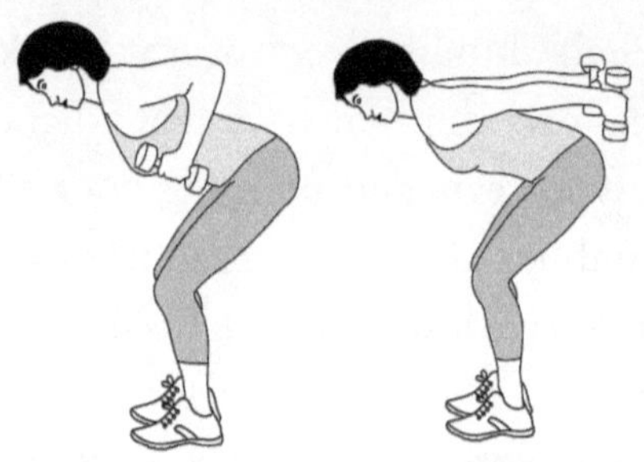

Tricep dip

Sit on the edge of the chair and hold tightly the edge of the chair at your side next to your hips. Extend your legs and your feet should be about hip-width apart with the heels touching the ground. Be comfortable in this position.

Then push steadily against your palms with some force to lift your body and slide forward just that your behind clears the edge of the chair. Move down until your elbows are bent between 45 and 90 degrees. Slowly push yourself back up to the start position slowly and repeat the movement 8–12 times.

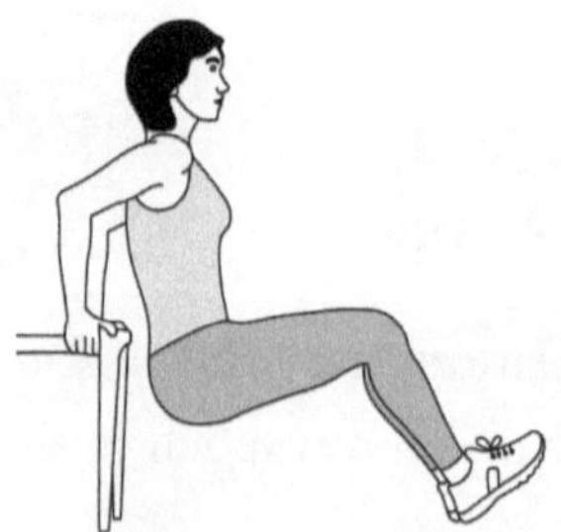

Smartphone Thumb

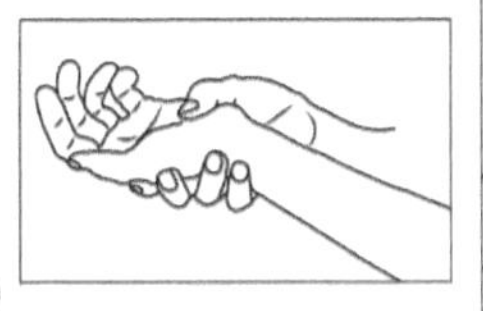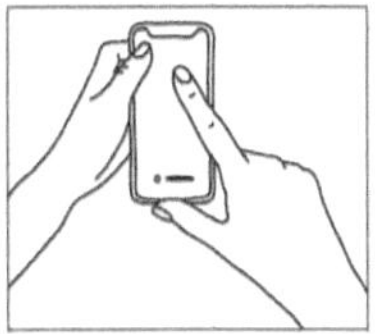

Cellphone neck, smartphone thumb, cellphone elbow are solely the tendinitis of neck, wrists, elbow or hands, out of which thumb is most vulnerable currently.

In our life smartphone today is a colossal, just as it toil a plethora of tasks. Even so, the human hand is not up until present evolved or metamorphosed to be harmonious with the apparatus.

Some time ago, I out-heard 'writers cramp' causing wrist pain which seems to me under no circumstances contrast to present times 'smartphone thumb' other than it arise from technology.

Throughout the time of using start phone, strained abnormal motion of bones in the thumb come about, inflaming the tendons of flexion and extension across the thumb and to the lateral side of your wrist. Initially it starts with displeasure at the base of right thumb, later pain and subsequently lock and outcry or stiffness befall in the morning.

Elderly are inclined to arthritis, shaping small bony knobs at the base of the thumb, middle joints and at the end of the joints of the fingers putting together ache, stiffness and numbness. In this context holding the smartphone incapacitate them. Despite not being previous arthritis, in youngsters also trapeziometacarpel joint osteoarthritis is reported causing pain in the upper limbs due to rise of new technologies.

Every mishap is a notice that something is wrong with methods, materials(object)- investigate them- then act.

The route to healing smart phone thumb, I'm telling, it's no new for all, but it's not serious yet unless with too much use of smart phone when you will become more regretful, then you will undeniably oblique this column of mine.

To prevent text thumb, use your forefingers for typing on the scores or use your voice to dictate message to alleviate typing.

Giving periodic breaks by putting your phone down can give the muscles and tendons relaxation.

Use "hunk and peck" style of typing where the phone is hold on one hand and the text is done with another or,

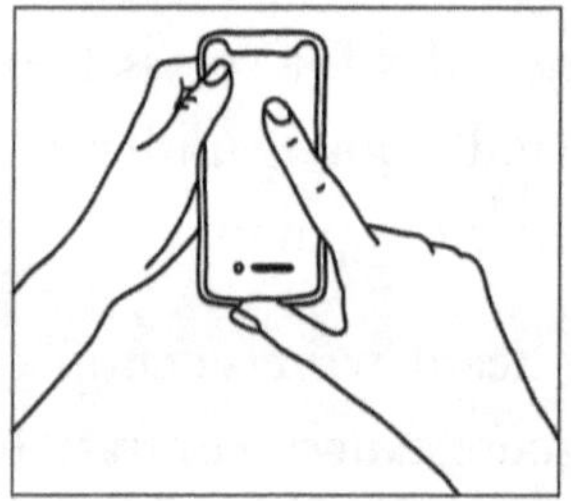

Use any comfortable position which doesn't need your wrist support and upright thumb, or just aim for- flexibility and strength.

Before going for exercises, I suggest warming up hands with gently massaging your hand and thereafter fomentation. But if your thumb is inflamed, apply ice or ice pack for 10–15 minutes.

Ball squeeze strengthener

For this exercise you can use soft gel stress relief ball or can go for yellow coloured smiley ball and grab it within your palms and squeeze as hard as you can for 3–5 seconds. Relax your grip slowly, repeat for 5–10 times.

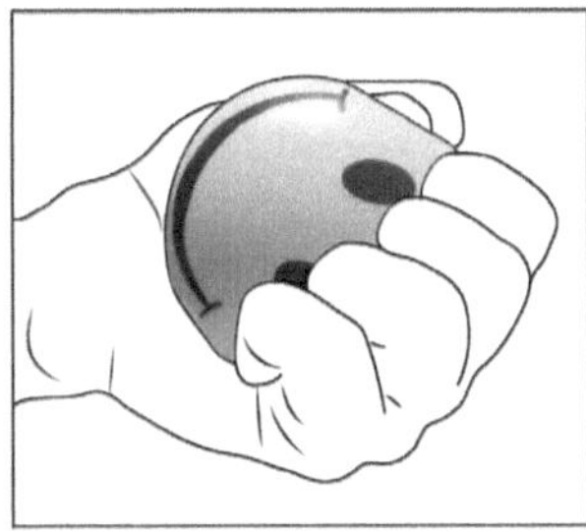

Hand grippers

Although these are the prime movers for the four digits other than thumb, you can use them to increase the strength of the hands.

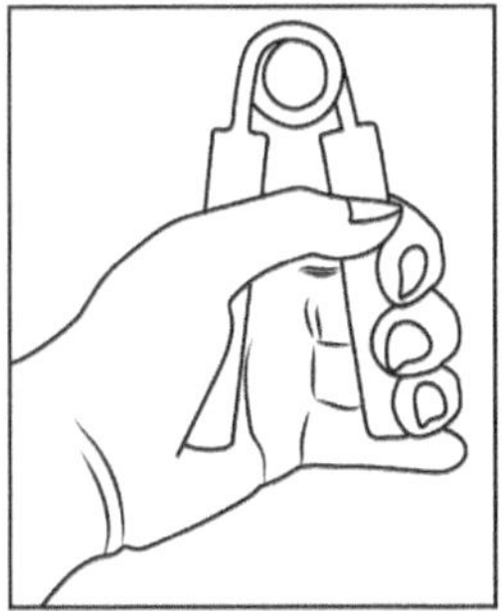

Further for increasing the range of motion, wrap your thumb across your fingers till you feel the stretch and then stretch your fingers wide apart again feeling the tension for stretch again.

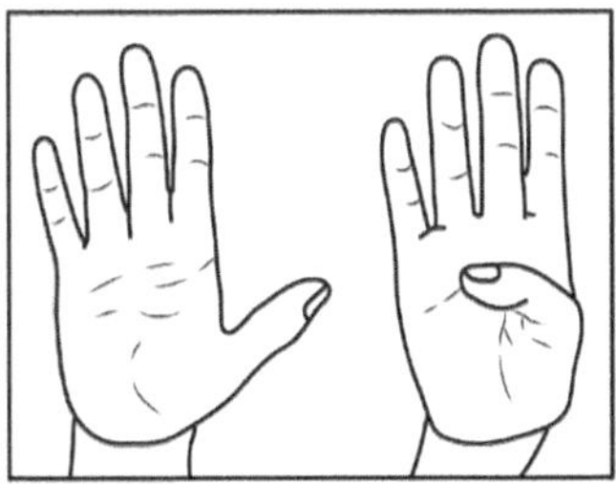

Making the fingers flexible would be easy by placing your flat palm on the flat surface and gently lifting every finger one by one and hold for around two seconds and then relax.

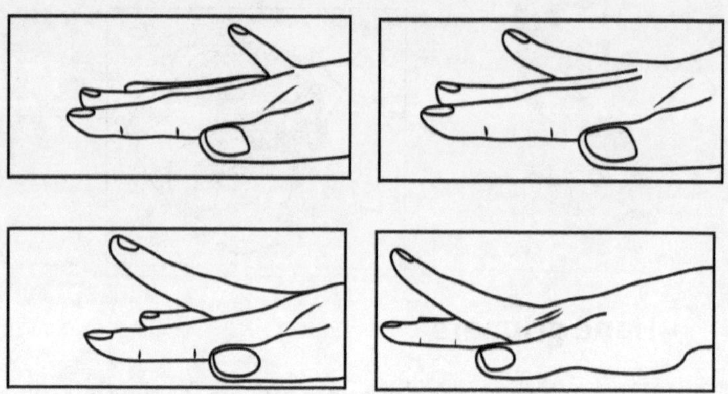

Remember if numbness, tingling, stiffness or inflammation continues do not hesitate to take the advice of doctor.

Cleavage Wrinkles

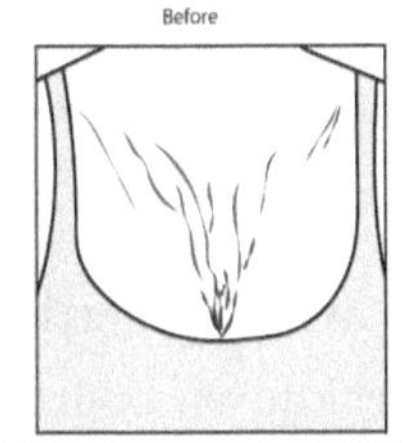
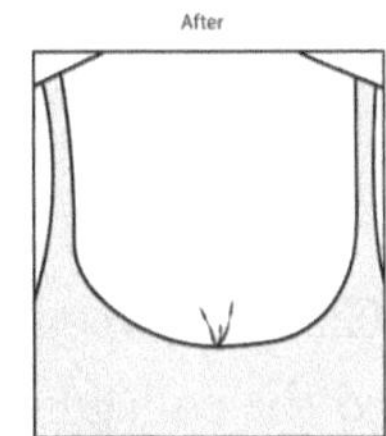

On the variety of my subject which is not like medical journal, but the gathered gradual concerns of women about aging and the straight easy ways to overcome it, I was writing in my own way to combat the ailments for what they are offering surgeries and botox.

It was not until the time, till I was not serious about the cleavage wrinkles, then happened when itself the cosmetologist showed her apprehension pertaining to her cleavage wrinkles.

It was the time, when I took my son to a cosmetologist to receive a treatment for acne. When we were waiting for our turn to get in, I just went through the hospital hoardings offering their speciality and amenities. This was the same time, I started writing, and it came to my notice that cosmetologist and I had one and the same intend to sustain aging malaise, where she is drawing upon surgeries and botox to combat the ailments, I have my own way to hold up.

As a beginner, trying my hand on pen, my intellectual curiosity botherlesly took me straight into her cabin and disclosed her my keynote with no excuse for fear of an apprehension whether she lend me her ears or not.

Surprisingly it happened, as if she was looking for an option for donning a camisole, she straight a way grilled me intense on her uneasy state of mind to hide her cleavage wrinkles. Despite being a cosmetologist, she insisted with authenticity opposition to botox for herself. Moreover was curious to catch up enticing alternatives rest of her natural life.

Although some woman would never grumble about cleavage wrinkles, other require to include this subject in my book, so I will be best to work it in last.

Cleavage wrinkles are deep vertical lingering furrow, seems absurd, is due to the collagen breakdown owing to aging. With this gravity pow the top breasts to a position that is afar than a body midline. Besides this those who spent hours wearing push up bra, sports bra, loiter or sleep for hours on one side, are prone to cleavage wrinkles.

Our unexpected sight go on our boobs only when we get off our bra in front of mirror in the bathroom before bathing, and if you have a sharp eye and if you are cautious about body then you might catch this inevitable creases on your chest. If this has not happened to you then it has to happen after reading this section, and just like me your focus will surly go on this unforeseen wrinkles, and in the first place you will also be exercised in front of mirror.

If you want a well formed cleavage without wrinkles, your center objective is supposed to be to engage in building chest muscles (Pectoralis major) which helps to raise your breasts thus giving perfect cleavage. Exercises like the bench press, push ups or the chest dip are a few that will help build your chest muscles. Using dumbbells will stimulate the muscle fibres in the mid-chest section that pull the breasts together and upwards.

Pretend to Fly

There's a lot of us out here that are birds, man. We all need to just fly. Just like the bird, extend your arms to the side, upto the shoulder level and move them as bird do when fly (up and down). Do the repetitions for certain time. This exercise certainly helps in building muscle strength of chest and shoulder, also give the breast somewhat of a lift and good cleavage subsequently.

Hand Pushes

This is my most loved isometric tension cleavage enhancing exercise. In this exercise you can develop tension in the muscle without contracting it. For this, make a prayer position of your hands. Then push the hand together against each other for about 5–10 seconds, repeat the exercise after 30 seconds, for some repetitions.

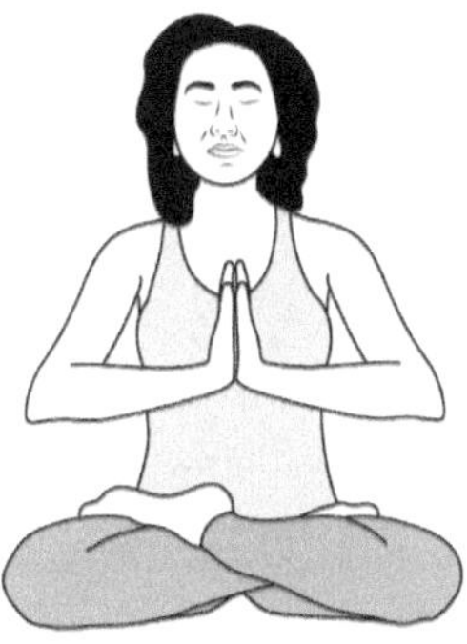

Wide Pushes

Wide pushups work distinctively other-than pushups and diamond pushups in its way it engage the biceps and the back muscles that stretch from your armpit to your spine. Here you don't have to change much your pushups, sheer keep your hands slightly wider than shoulder-width apart, with fingers slightly outward and bend your elbows out to the sides to lower torso toward the floor where the chest does not touch the chest muscles.

Instead on toes you can try this exercise on lying on your knees also. Do 8–15 reps. Try 3 sets.

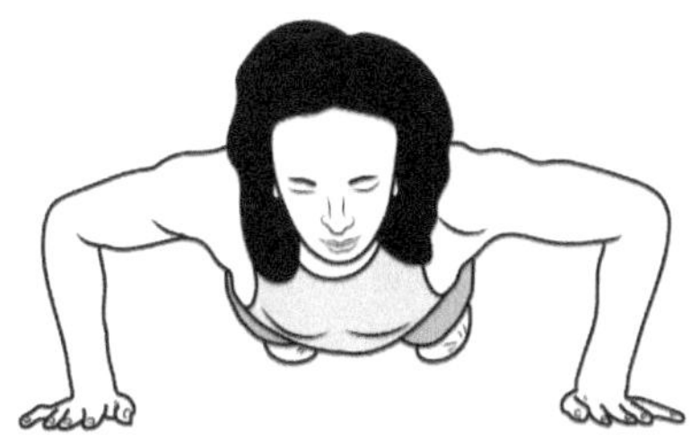

Affix Your Sleeping Position

There will be many of you who sleeps on the same side on the night, get herself in the morning on the same side. Very well, this sign probably can be the indicator of deep sleep when the body and mind ties them together with the golden chain, but think, sleeping 6–7 hours on the same side will not invite creases between your breasts form the oppression of breasts? which with age will progress toward being more permanent. Therefore, initiate a useful sleeping habit for yourself like sleeping on your back more prolonged relative to sleeping on your side.

Massage

As we age, oxygen levels in the skin cells naturally decreases, shun the skin less elastic allowing fine lines and wrinkles to appear. Till hell freezes over skin needs oxygen in assisting to repair the regeneration of collagen and elastin tissue. Many oxygen boost skin creams are being publicised in market for doing your chase. Don't sacrifice, gift your chest skin with good oxygen boost by stimulating the blood flow to the area by massaging with oil over your chest and around breasts in circular motion, at least once in a week.

Bra Bulge

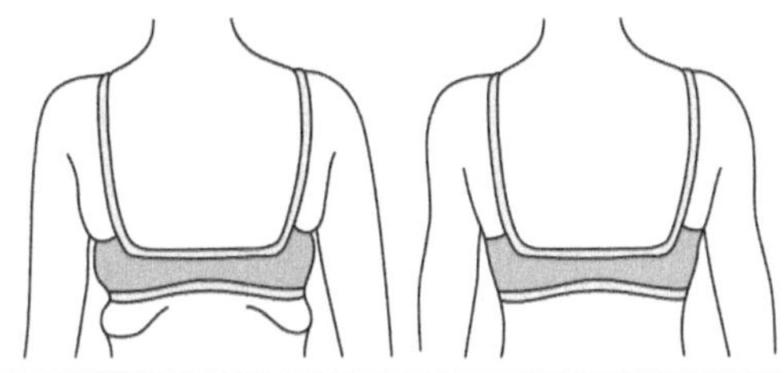

Like many unending issues, back fat is also ignored as late as it goes into surge around and picks out from around your bra, which every woman must have grappled with in the form of awkward double boob, side boob and back fat, someday. And once it outstretch, our trail to knock the bulge begins. Although for some it seems appealing, it may be able to taint your figure and wear yourself to a frazzle. Here earliest action should be taken otherwise this surplus broad bun of adipose tissue which seems to me like phantom resist the admirable change.

During the transit through tricenarian, quadragenarian, quinquagenarian and so on women get less physically active, there is decline in ovarian production of steroidal hormone resulting in weight gain and change in fat distribution. Also metabolism slows down much rapid in menopause leading to reduction in muscle mass and increase in weight around the back, nearly in all women in one of the norm as it could be upper back fat (which dislodge over the back of the bra strap), mid back fat (which ride near the back of the waist) and lower back top fat (that overhang over the head of the pants).

Ladies, our breast size is instrumental in the architecture of our persona perhaps could be one of the reason for bra bulge. I personally endorse optimum breast size complimenting the physique for solely at first even I also can't hang in round the clock the oppressions and notches of bra belt on my shoulder to hold big breasts and secondly, viewing the connect of big breasts with risk of breast cancer.

If you have to overcome this fright, your aim should be to strengthen the back muscles because back muscles not only reshape your back also helps to improve posture and the taller appearance makes you look instantly thinner and raise your confidence.

Superman pose

To fitter back make a 'superman' pose by lying on your stomach and slowly lift both your arms and legs simultaneously as much as possible. Hold this position for as long as you comfortably can and keep looking straight ahead.

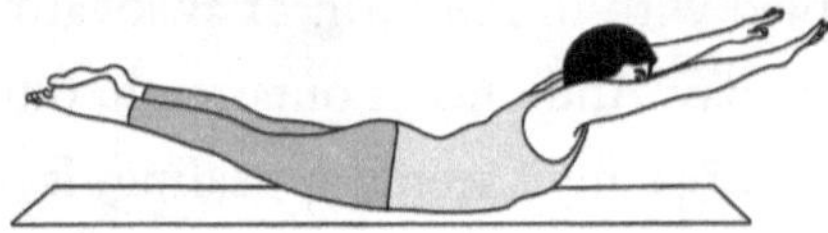

Aqua-man pose

Equivalent to 'superman' you can go for 'aqua-man'. For that first lift your right arm and the left leg as good as you can. And when you lower the two down, lift your left arm and your right leg. Do these movements with all possible haste.

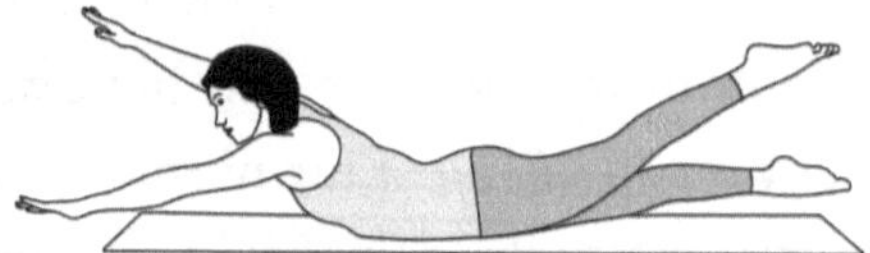

Squats

Squats are not new to us. We unknowingly squat many a time during cooking, going to toilet, etc. But when it comes to exercise you have to adopt a proper technique. Since squats isometrically use both the lower and upper back, moving the hips back, bend the knees and hips to lower the torso and after halting for a few seconds longer, return to the upright position. Remember keep your back straight with a slight forward tilt while moving. If you go down quickly it can put pressure on your knees. To avoid knee injuries rotate your knees internally while lowering your body and externally while rising.

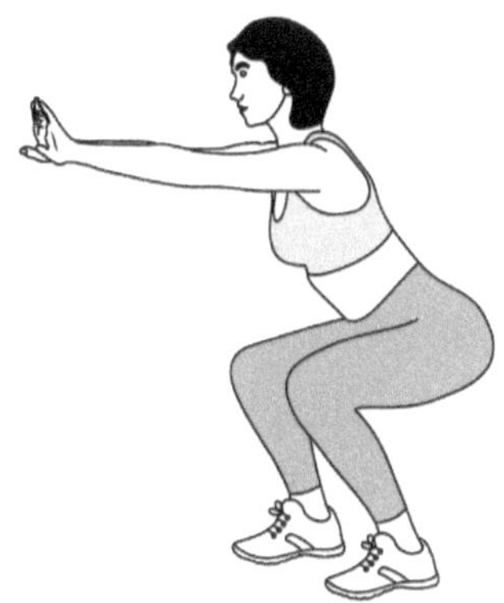

Pull-ups and pushups

Pull-ups and pushups are simple low impact timeless exercises that works for the complete upper body and can be performed virtually anywhere. Besides strengthening the muscular system, it even helps in making your nervous system stronger.

If you want to set home gym at home then you can build your own pull up bar out of the many types like ceiling-mounted, wall-mounted, door-frame, free standing pull-up bars and floor mounted; if its possible go for any, otherwise I think wall mounted push up bars are safer, you can add chin-up bars, lateral pulley bar, tricep bar, roller pull and extension chain.

Catch hold of the bar with you palms facing away from you and your body extended. Now slowly pull yourself up until your chin reaches above the bar. The only difference between pull-ups and chin ups is of holding the bar. For chin ups, you grip the bar with your palms facing you and in pull- ups you flip the bar with your palms facing away from you.

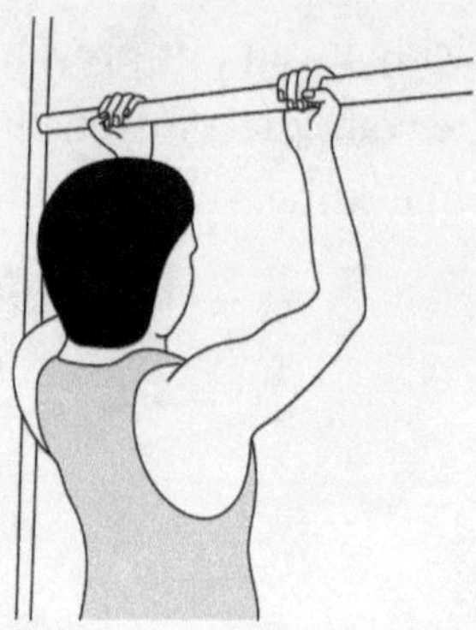

Swimmers who are helpless amid lockdown can fake it like you are swimming into deep water moving yourself in squat posture and drag water resistance.

And even if you have no desire to exercise at all, thats not a problem either. Overlong the activity that pleases you like Zumba, running, yoga, aerobics. In any way you want nothing doing, go for well shaped bra that has a broad back band and thick straps to rescue you form this pesky bra bulge.

Saggy Breasts

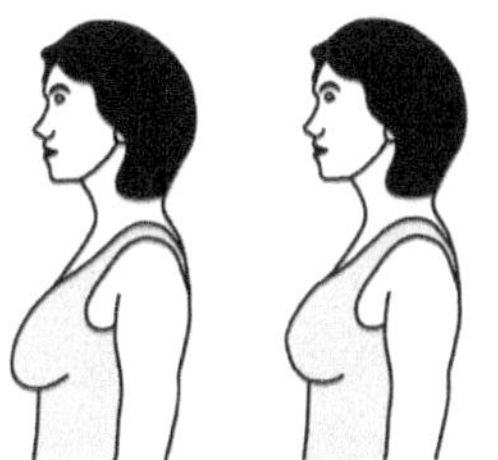

In many of powwow a solitary concealed interrogation come along- Why do woman flash on her breast size? While there are many friction of opinions, just to be peaceful over scuffle I say-beauty lies in the eyes of beholder and not in the breasts you happen to be holding. Whereas my hidden consciousness always delight me of nicely shaped breasts.

Even so this state doesn't remain the same all along the woman's life, her breasts will take leave from its position and wane. Although this tends to be the universal cosmetic change woman forbids saggy breasts.

Separating the frequently asked questions about 'the prospects of lifting saggy breasts', it was in my drop dead list, but to take the edge off anxiety and distress my answer could be both 'yes' and 'no'.

For the reply of 'no' to lifting the destined saggy breasts- don't spend your precious hours fearing the inevitable, for many things influence breasts shape and size right from your pregnancies, genetic predisposition, hormonal changes and to some degree it's an essential feature of aging where the glandular tissue that produce breast firmness succumb to gravity and somewhat sag, while in most advanced stage the nipples are dropped down the fold and takes aim towards the ground. So, you can't do much to prevent sagging rather confess ageing, gracefully.

Anatomy says that breasts don't have the muscles, so how can you firm the breast tissue with exercise? Hence learning to love your soulmate no matter what size she is and enjoying each others asset on its own terms, just think how many industries would go out of business.

..........and for the 'yes' side, apart from surgical method of breast augmentation I would suggest to work on strengthening the pectoralis muscles beneath the breasts, for adding muscle is almost acting like a push-up bra, giving an illusion of bigger and slightly lifted breasts.

Wide Pushups

Out of many exercises, as I told you earlier wide pushups are easy to do at home and still more effective in the sense it also improves lean muscle mass, your bone health and also your confidence. If you have any former wrist injury or you are getting wrist pain while doing, go for an alternative of forearm pushups or knuckle pushups.

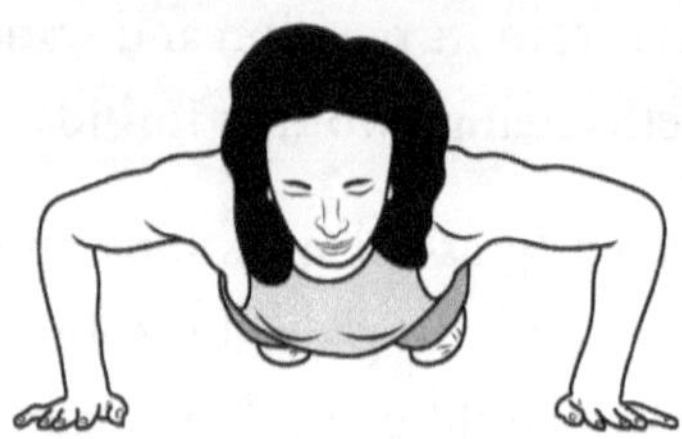

Wall Pushups

While I'm in kitchen, my inner woman hold onto the front wall relentlessly halfway my cooking and pick up some fix for the best loved and effortless choice of wall pushups on the way of burning calories and muscle building.

Stay behind 2–3 feet from the wall and put your palms on it shoulder-width apart. While inhaling, bend your elbows and get closer to the wall. While returning back to the starting position exhale and make sure your abs are tight and glutes squeezed. Try 3 sets of 10 repetitions and the 30 second break after each set.

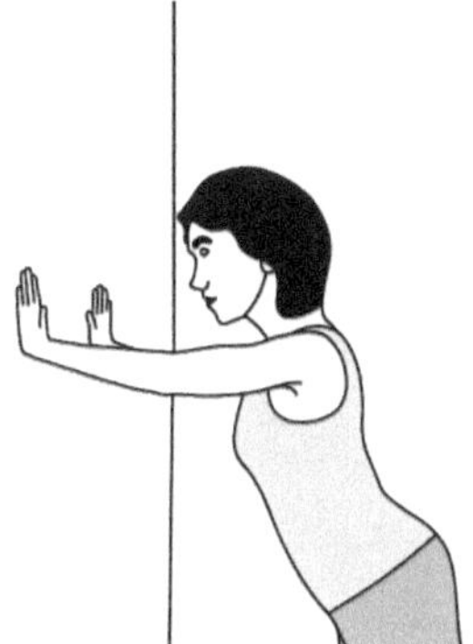

Cobra-Pose

To start my day right, I set off my day in my bed by virtue of "cobra-pose" to praise God for our well being and also as a light morning warmup.

Clear the bedding, lay on your stomach with your legs extended, make sure the top of your legs are resting on your bed. Place your hands under your shoulders with the elbows ticked in. Start lifting your head and chest off the ground while drawing your shoulders back-try to straighten your arms as much as you can. Hold this position for 30 seconds for 3 times while taking 5 second break.

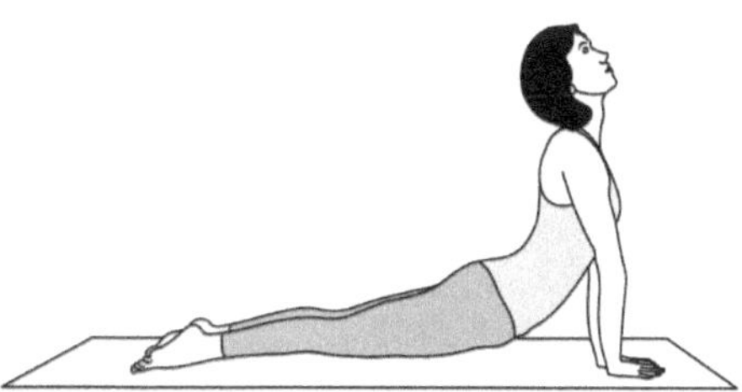

Prayer Position

Here comes my favourite pose again. To gift your breast a well-defined outline, sit in Indian style with your legs crossed, the soles of your feet facing the ceiling and heals pressing against your abdomen. Thereafter join your hands together between your breasts (prayer position) with both elbows slightly raised. Gently squeezing and relaxing both palms together make contraction in the breasts, making the outer curve of breast defined.

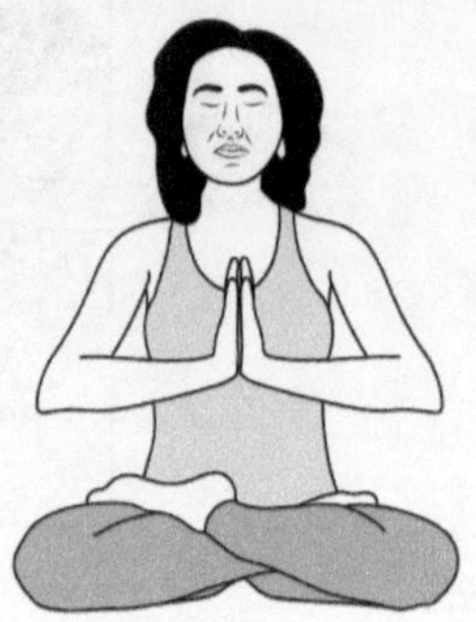

Massage

Massaging around the outside, bottom and inner areas of the breasts may help stimulate the lymph vessels and could prevent or reduce lymphedema in the arms and chest.

Finally yet important, I ask every women to go for self breast examination at regular intervals to detect early breast cancer.

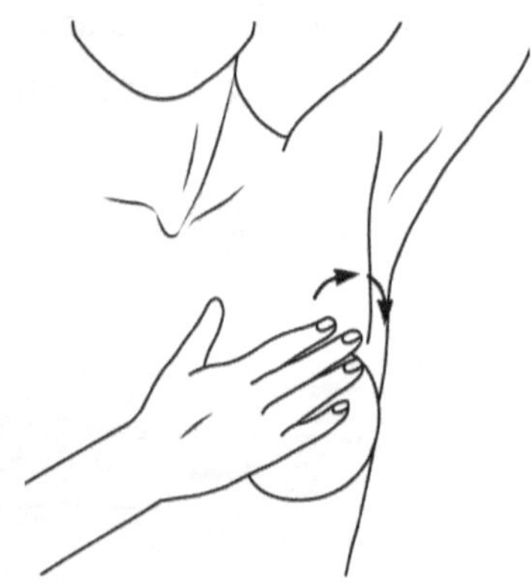

Middle Age Spread

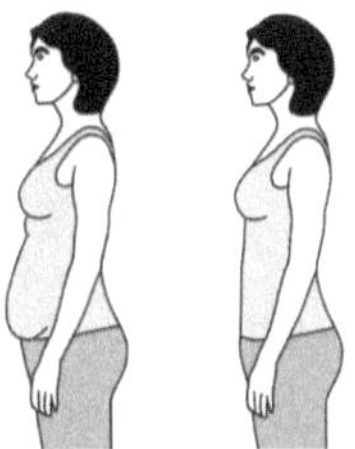

When my two brothers and I had our own's sweet time with my mother, we swung around all over the place to hold her extended belly which comes across as chucklesome mushy-cushy float and my mummy used to find great pleasure in saying "I owned this asset of three children", with a sense of achievement, undermining the belly fat.

Graciously that fact was the earlier familiar motherhood tune which I think every mother got acclimated with. But with the advent of time, no mother bring about a wish to settle upon this hanging belly killing her figure.

In eighties this abdominal obesity is emphasised first when a connection of belly fat is sought with metabolic disorders causing cardiac dysfunction just after general obesity.

So, there is no reason to anticipate this "baker's dozen" as destined, rather this middle age spread should be of greater concern because as people live through middle years the share of fat to their body weight increases, for that reason their waistline widens.

Out of the two types of belly fat, the 'abdominal fat' is easy to assess by holding them in two fingers whereas on the other hand the 'visceral fat' which contributes to about 10% is far flung mysterious, hidden headrest between the abdominal organs.

Whatever the circumstances of your body shape, excess fat around a specific location isn't a big deal for your health and per annum pleads the evidence that the visceral fat is more hazardous for it increases the risk of diabetes, breast cancer, heart attacks, stroke, colorectal cancer, Alzheimer's than the fat which you can pinch with your fingers.

After hoarding a lot bits and pieces, at this point, I figure out more dominance of 'belly fat theory' over 'body fat theory'. So putting primacy of 'belly fat theory' on top, which says that abdominal fat cells are biologically active and therefore its appropriate to think particularly abdominal fat cells as endocrine gland or organ producing hormones and has their effects on body shape and fat distribution. From below I want you individually to earmark your problem area /shortcomings and determine the best exercise and life style changes to shape up.

TYPE OF BELLY	APPEARANCE	CAUSES	MANAGEMENT
Adrenal belly	Fat accumulates around waist leading to saggy waist. Associated with fatigue, back-pain, poor memory, sleep problems, nervousness.	Increased levels of cortisol	Prioritise mindfulness and meditation, gentle yoga, proper sleep
Thyroid belly	Accumulation of belly fat around the waistline, weight gain in the upper and lower body simultaneously. Associated hair loss, saggy underarm skin, brittle finger nails, cold extremities	less thyroid hormone	Treat hypothyroidism by medicines, exercises like walking, jogging, biking, dancing, push-ups, sit-ups, abdominal crunches, leg squats

Ovary belly	Saddle bags and lower stomach fat. Additionally thin hairs, bloating, frequent acne outbreaks, heavy periods, facial hairs, ovarian cysts, headaches	Excess of oestrogen hormone	Balance your hormone levels, if necessary by medications. Add diet that is rich in protein, and fat from vegetable sources and low in animal origin
Liver belly	Abdomen seems like pot, arms and legs rather thin. Also bloating, digestive problem, back pain, soreness	Decreased production or impaired release of bile	Add more portions and reduce complex carbohydrates (peas, beans, whole grains and vegetables) from your diet. Avoid alcohol, soda

In consonance with above belly you can pick up your own type and can head accordingly to reduce belly fat, somewhat partly.

Out of the leading questions related to assessing health measures pertaining to belly fat, the formula for measuring it, the normal measurements, its limitations, conflicting information and other criss-cross questions confusing your intellect, I would say everybody's constitution is different plus these health measures is only a standard measurement of the average female, apart from this there's plenty of factors that need to count as well.

One of the simplest way, although I feel that it's not absolutely fair but still if you want to roughly consider the risk related indicators of your health by your own at home, one of the simplest way by which you can easily keep an eye on your fat counts and body fat mass and predict your health related to overweight including heart disease, fertility, etc; is by measuring your waist circumference and waist- hip ratio.

You will be sceptical while reviewing belly fat, how I'm talking about waist, hips. That's because, after counting, if your waist comes more than your hips, it acknowledges that much fat is accumulated around your belly which is conclusive for 'intra abdominal obesity',which is dangerous than your butt, thighs, arms, etc., and is applied to probability of heart diseases, hypertension, diabetes, etc. The lessened the better.

Furthermore 'waist-hip ratio' show good correlation with body fat as measured by the most accurate. Weight-related risk is measured in three ways-

Waist- hip ratio

Place a measuring tape around your waist in line with your naval, don't suck in your stomach, breath out normally.

If you are a women than waist circumference over 35 inches is considered high risk, the measurement between 31.6 to 34.9 inches are at intermediate risk. If you are measuring in centimetre, 80–87 cm is intermediate risk and circumference above 88cm is considered high risk.

Measure the waist circumference as above;

Measure the hips at their widest point, which is usually around where your thigh meets your hips and the lower part of your hip joint out to your side. Divide your waist size by your hip size and interpret your result.

Waist-to-hip ratio chart

Health risk	Women
Low	0.80 or lower
moderate(healthy)	0.81–0.85
High	0.86 or higher

Women should have waist to hip ratio under 1.0-o.90 or lower. According to WHO having a WHR of over 1.0 may increase the risk of developing conditions that relate to being overweight, including even when BMI are in normal range.

Having higher WHR means there is more fat in the middle of you, that gives "apple" shape to the body and signifies greater risk of certain health condition other than "pear" shape (hips>upper body)

In general, woman do not mind being their underweight, healthy weight, because she always considers herself fat and which is their status quo, just somehow try anyway to reduce it. Here is a tool to measure your obesity i.e. BMI, which fairly detects your healthy weight for your height but unfair on to detect body fat, muscle mass or bone density.

Irrespective of your body types and ages, BMI can be measured from the following equation-

weight(kg)/height(m) = BMI.

Interpret your result-

BMI	Weight status
Below18.5	Underweight
18.5–24.9	Normal or healthy weight
25.0–29.9	Overweight
30.0 and above	Obese

Indians are not very heavy built as Americans or other heavy weight genes, hence a lower BMI accepted as normal is 23 (https://care.diabetesjournals.org>co...).

Seeing your weight status you be cautious on your own, next, why and how much you have to be aware of your health and risks associated with it.

For burning subcutaneous fat it is necessary to burn energy in the form of calories. So, you can go for running, jumping rope which is like winning half the battle. Next you can strengthen abdominal muscles to flaunt your flat belly.

To add variations to increase fat burning power, involve running for 1 minute followed by two minute walk, then go for another 2 minute running or go for intense jumping rope.

Walking at a brisk pace for about 30–45 minutes four or five days every week or more will also work. Avoid brisk walking on the rough bump surface.

If you are not having any knee or lumber pain, you can go for skipping which works on your transverse abdominus, rectus abdominus and your inner and outer obliques.

Burpee

If you have a keen pulsating desire to lose your gut, you need to work as many muscles as possible of shoulders, hips, back, core, arms etc., and burpee does just that. It involves going from a push up position to a jump and back to push up position. Be cautious while hoping through these positions. Maintain the proper push up position. Try a basic burpee, you remain in the raised plank with your core contracted and back straight, and then jump your feet back towards your hands and shoulders directly over your hands as shown in figure then round off the move by leaping onto the air with your arms straight above you(as in figure). Be aware, don't stomp loud heavy step after jump. It's possible you get breathless after one burpee: do one burpee, as fast as you can, then take one deep breath at the top and loosen your hands, body and relax on the way down. While doing you can get pressure on your ankles, knees and wrists. Therefore don't forget to do some warm up before and stretching after the workout. Gradually increase the counts.

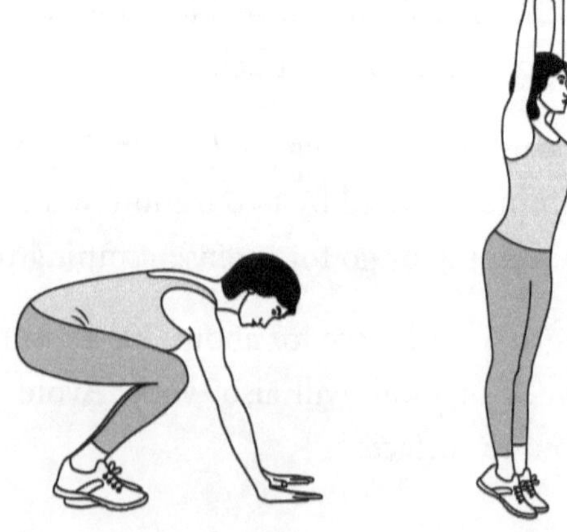

Stomach Crunch

Is the more direct way to target abdominal muscles and to burn the belly fat without any equipment.

Lying flat on your back, knees bent and feet even on the floor, hip-spaced apart, place your hands on your thighs, over your chest or behind your ears.

Slowly bend up towards your knees until your shoulders are about 3 inches off the floor without yanking your head off the floor. Hold the position for a few seconds and lower down slowly. With regular practice you will definitely clamp your stomach muscles and feel the difference. Perform 10–12 stomach crunches in each set of three with a gap of 30 seconds .

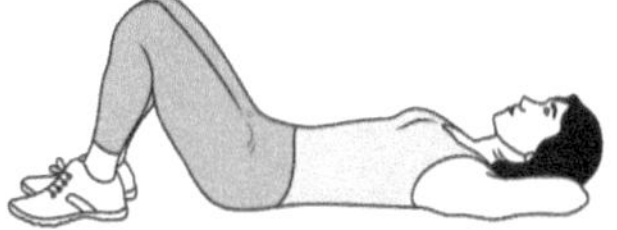 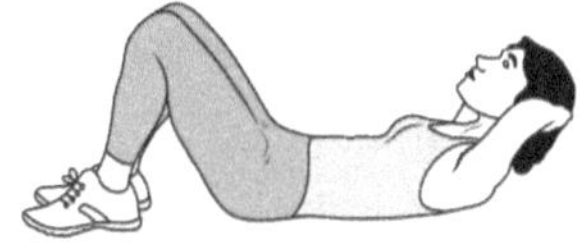

Oblique Crunch

While doing abdominal exercises your obliques and deep transverse abdominal muscles are neglected, oblique crunch better target these.

Lie on your side with forearm down and knees slightly bent. Take the top hand behind your head. Confirm your position in mirror. Now lift both the legs jointly and bring your knees to your elbow while the same time crunch your elbows towards your knees as shown in figure. Also squeeze your waistline. Complete 12–15 repetitions and switch sides.

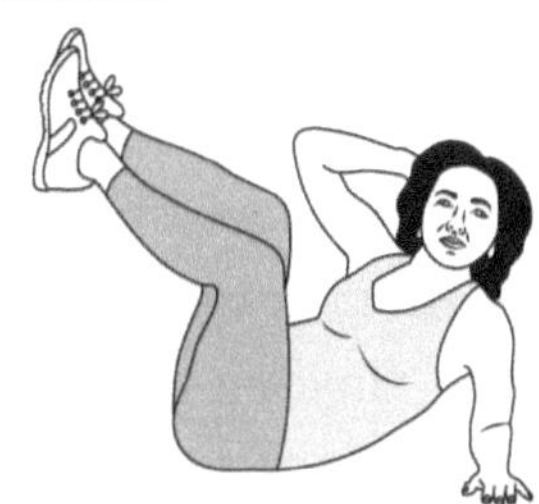

Plank

Plank is one of the best exercises that targets lower back and core muscles, builds your isometric strength, improves your posture.

Lie on your front propped up on your forearms and toes. Keep your legs straight and hips raised to create a straight and rigid line from head to toe.

Your shoulders should be directly above your elbows. Focus on keeping your abs contracted during the exercise. Hold this position for 5 to 10 seconds and repeat 8 to 10 times. To make it easy, you can perform your plank with your knees on the floor. Remember, look down (don't raise your head) and don't allow your back to sink during the exercise. If you are in it, you can hold this position for longer time and could feel the stretch. Remember, if you have any problem related to your back, lumber or knees, first consult your doctor.

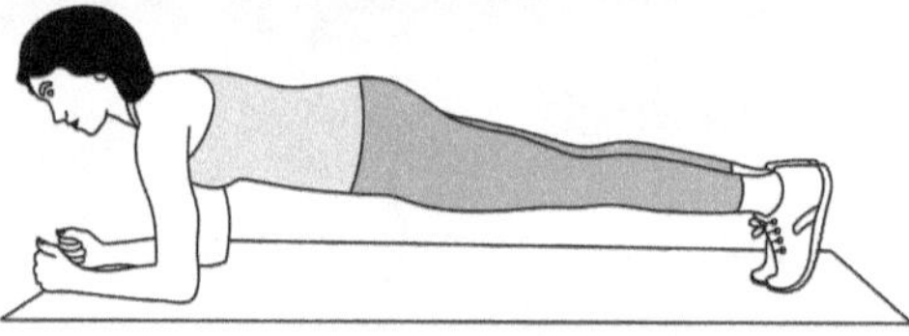

Side plank

Lie on your right side with your legs straight and feet hold up on top of each other. Place your right elbow under your right shoulder with your forearm denoting away form you and make the fist of your hand .

With your neck neutral, exhale and support your core. Start going your hips off the ground with an aim to support your weight on your elbow and the side of your right foot. Body should be straight alongside, don't let the lower back sink. Cling to for the duration of this position. Aim between 15–60 seconds. Repeat on your left side. For ease you can even perform with your knees on the floor

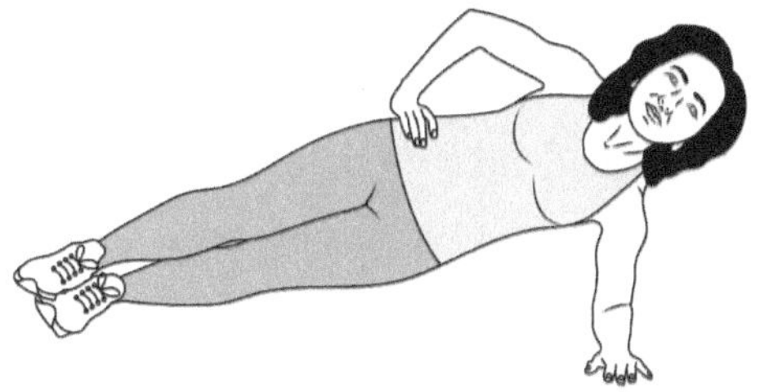

Squats

Are the high intensity compound movement which not only targets largest muscle groups—like your glutes, quadriceps and hamstrings—also targets your rectus abdominus, obliques, transverse abdominus and erector spinae. If you are pressed for time, you can break your session into morning and evening. When you have a good form, you can add weights like dumbbells, kettle bells in a low carry position. Next try dumbbell shoulder squat using light weights.

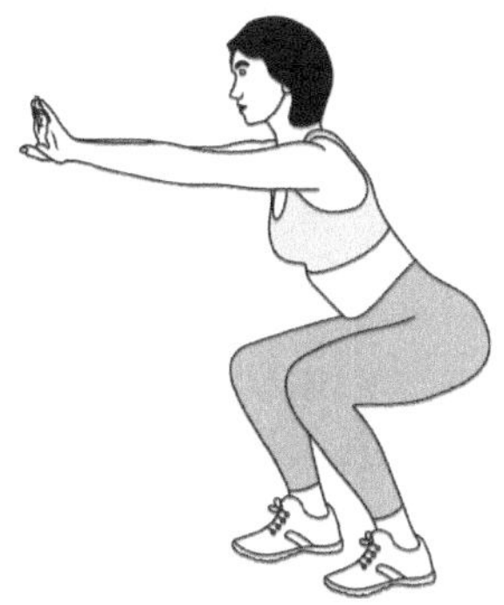

Stomach vacuum

Stomach vacuum is a great effortless technique to train abdominal muscles for great posture and reduce belly fat. As long as sun's rays do not burn until brought to focus, identically to make the most of this exercise you have to accentuate your breathing.

Concentrating all your thoughts on work, stand vertical on the floor and place your hands on your hips. Now, exhale all the air out, as much you can achieve. To good effect, you should sense there is no air in your lungs. Thereafter inhale and swell your chest, and take your stomach to the extend possible. Then, exhaling move to touch your naval to the backbone. Initially try to hold this position for few seconds and gradually increase for more seconds, and release slowly. This completes one contraction. Repeat 10 times for one set.

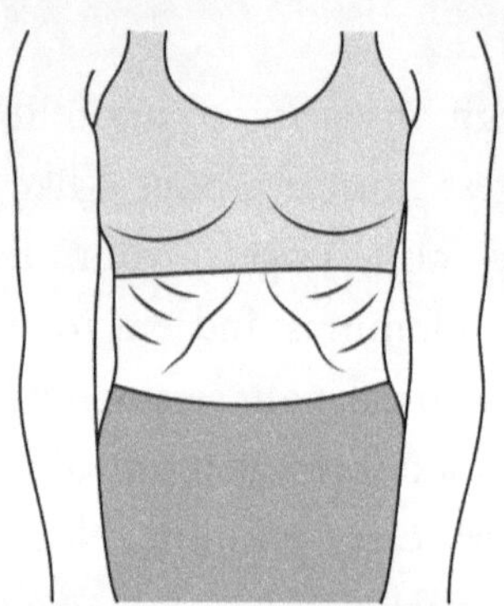

One of the international journal of environmental research and public health quoted that the exposure to sunlight in animals could lead to a reduction in weight gain and metabolic function and its review highlights that few studies have looked at the effects of sunlight in humans, in regards to weight gain. If we take these clues and make an attempt to do it regularly, which is effortless and that too without charge; so what's wrong with it.

While studying all of our dietary habits, I found that the most unhealthiest thing on your plate is your stuffs like all packed baking mixes which contains trans fat added to increase its shelf lives, little less is a carb dense foods, fried foods, processed food, spicy food, raw vegetables, alcohol, dairy products, acidic foods. If we rate all these then your plate will be empty. Then I will just ask you to pay attention to it, making little effort to reduce its use can be confirmed.

"Ideal" Shape Up

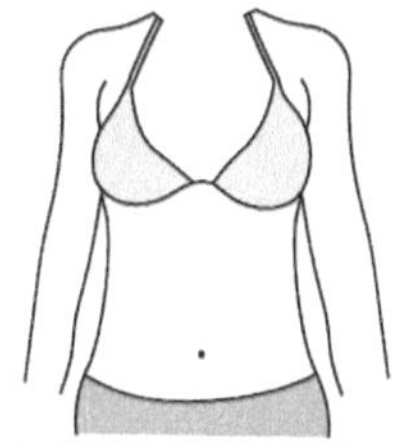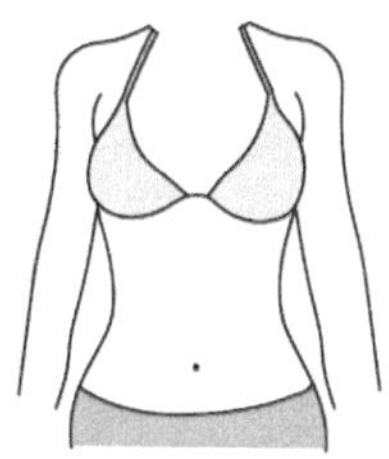

Referring at the nude sculptures of the masters all over the civilisation, it seems like curves have been the idle precision of the chiselers- those women have cosmic standard of beauty and a quantum of female attractiveness.

Even today, gazing a curvaceous women can long for honor in the grey matter of men. But they forget, beautiful women comes in all shapes and sizes, regular widespread bracket are like rectangle, triangle or "pear" shaped, inverted triangle or "apple" shaped and hourglass. To a significant extent women has infatuation for hourglass although it doesn't seem to be realistic, still to tempt you the industry is always endeavouring to create the illusion of hourglass.

Although the measurements of hourglass figure are 36–24–36 or 90–60–90 it does not mean you should fit into it as one cannot change the basic body you are born with. Rather than striving for this "ideal" I insist to find motivation in getting stronger, fitter or healthier.

The main crux of balanced beauty is proportion your bust, waist and hips, with enough even well-defined waistline. Those who do not have, don't rush to. Instead, duly get hold of the affair, aim for optimum overall health, break the rules and sculpt ideal body for own.

While researching on body shape, health and perceptions of beauty, I can conclude to round off the waists size that should be visibly narrower than the hips which bear a resemblance to the lower curve of hourglass who draws regard as similar with waist-hip ratio.

To sculpt your muscles and round your curves you will have to tone from all over ie. butt, thighs, shoulder, triceps and core (rectus abdominis, transverse abdominis, internal and external obliques).

Forearm Plank

As it trims your tummy also arm in arm work for your curves.

Take a kneeling position. Bend your elbows to 90 degree and thrust forward to place your hands and forearms on the floor. Divide your kneeling weight in your hands by spreading your fingers apart. Be stable, keep your body straight and keep your abdominal muscles tight. Hold this position for as long as you can do. Repeat. With practice you can challenge further with knee to floor, palms up, side plank, single-leg plank, single-arm plank.

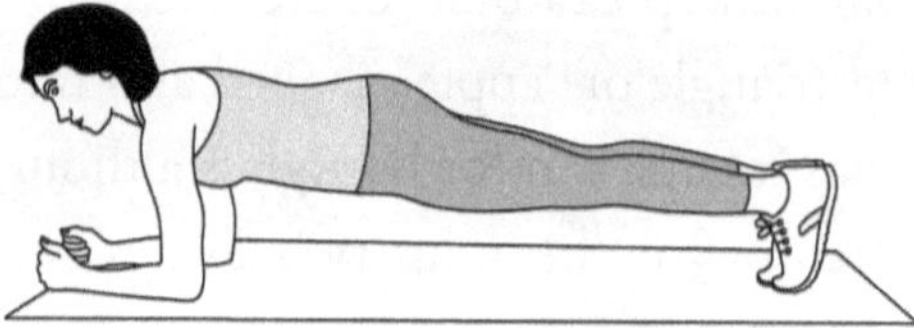

Plank Toe Tap

This is the easiest version of dynamic plank. Start in a push-up position. lift one foot to tap to the side about 12 inches from your stationary foot, hold it for 30 seconds and then return, alternating feet. Repeat.

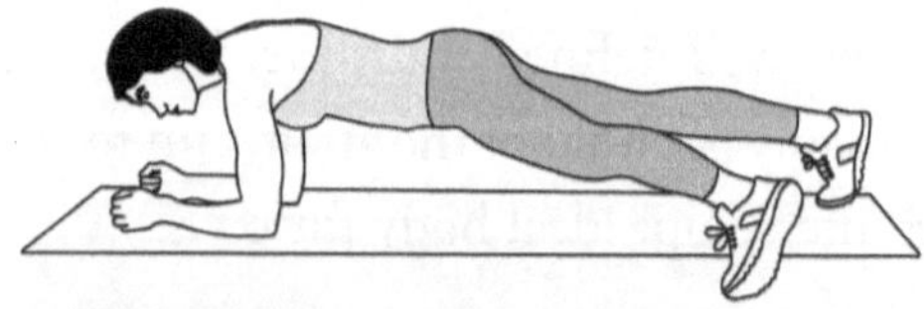

Alternating Arm Raise

Begin with kneeling position, raise your right arm and left leg up off the ground, keeping your upper body stable, hold for few seconds, come back to starting position. Repeat for left hand and right leg. Add more repetitions further.

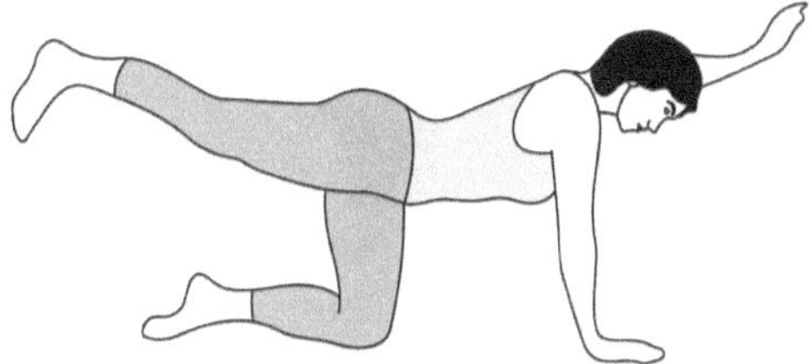

Mermaid Crunch

It may seem little hard but I think with practice it will work best for your obliques. To sculpt your obliques lie on your left side with your left arm bent, supporting your upper body and your right arm behind your head. Lift your legs about a foot off the frowns, this is your starting position. Keeping your feet together draw your knees and right elbow to meet over your torso then extend your legs back to start. Do eight repetition on the right side, then repeat on left side.

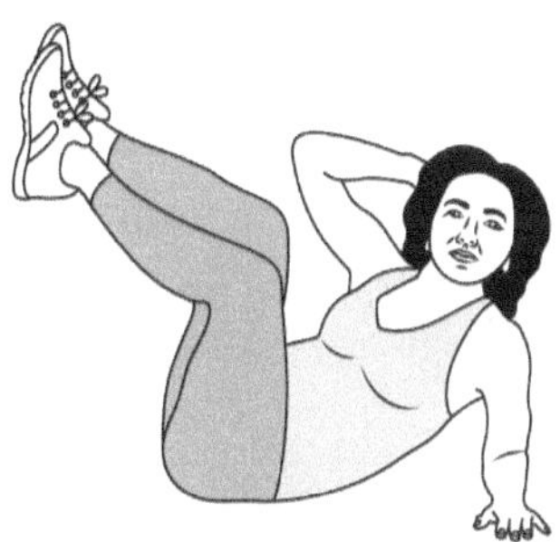

Tai Chi Lunges

To tone your butts, thighs and core-stand with your feet-width part, extend your arms straight out in front of you and palms facing down. Now, towards your right side take a huge step making a good balance, bending your right knee until its bent from 45 degree to 90 degree (make sure to keep your knee from extending over your toes). Stay in this side-lunge position and by rotating your waist, rotate your torso and outstretched arms to the left. Come back to the center and then to the starting position, next go for the opposite side.

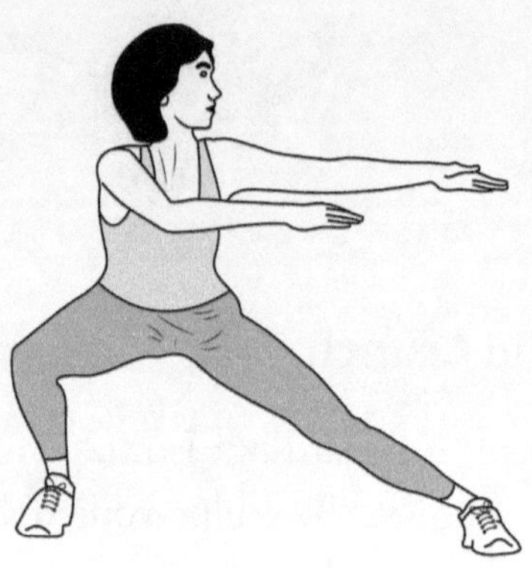

Lateral Lunges

Lunges are fantastic lower body exercises works on glutes medius (a muscle on the outer edge of your hip),outer thighs(lateral quads), inner thighs. Stand tall with your feet parallel and shoulder width apart. Your back should be straight and your weight on heels. Take a big step to the side and, ensuring you keep your torso as upright as possible, lower until the knee of your leading leg is bent at around 90 degree keeping your tailing leg straight. Push back up and return to the starting position.

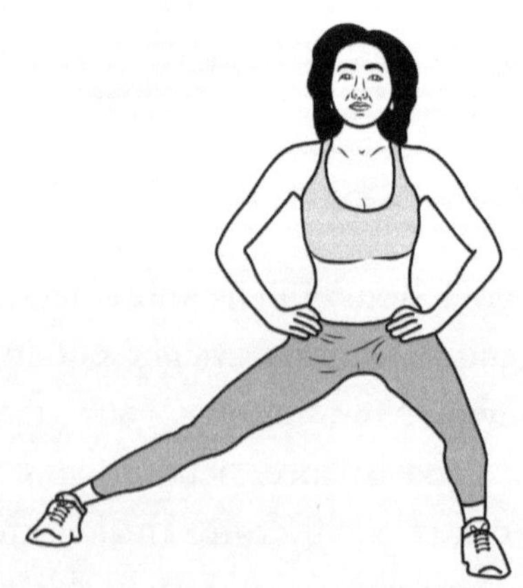

Cardio Routine

A good many ladies do not find time for workouts and it is also true. But if you yourself think for a moment in your mind then in less time than you expected can finish your workout to burn calories and drop pounds. like you can split your cardio into smaller workouts a day. In particular-you can exercise for at least 15–20 minutes in the morning before starting your home routines, you can take a 10 minute walk after your lunch break in the office and at night you can walk for 15–20 minutes. Or make anything possible according to your wish, for instance-jogging, bicycling, power walking, swimming and aerobics. Any of these activities may be appropriate to burn the overall fat and tone, streamline the abdominal muscles.

Love Handles

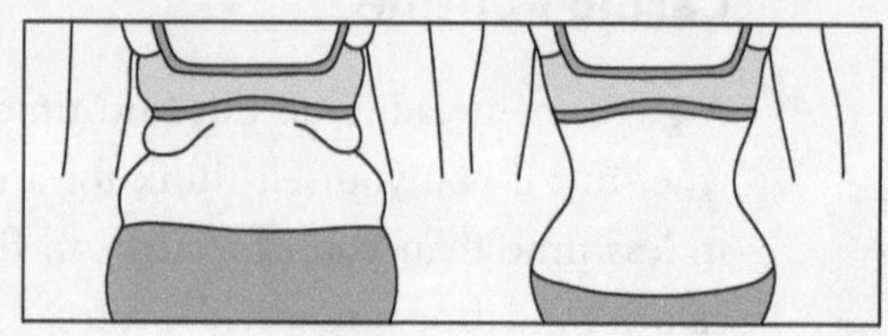

In the clash of opinions or ideas of "love" in their name, you see, there is no way to love these handles. Even so, I love these handles for its glorious position on top of the obliques.

You see, I often wonder why this term gets "criticism" for as much as love handles are the excess fat that sits at the side of your waist and over hangs. But having it doesn't confined you on the way to fat. Well, it's hard to regret that our side fat exists in some degree because of utter physiology and not merely food.

Love handles aren't dangerous, but they may indicate underlying risk factors for chronic illness includes blood pressure, high cholesterol, breathing issues, osteoarthritis, liver diseases…or if killing your looks. So, it's imperative to get rid off this muffin top since the fat around the butt, thigh is stubborn as a mule and take hell of time to go away unless this studded fat doesn't go into the blood stream to get oxidised and make energy.

For me love handles have highest regard as it stands foremost in love making and doesn't harbor the ounce of muscles. But requires the highest struggles, if they dollop over your pants or make your dresses bulge. Here, to eventually shed the omnipresent pockets of fat your initial goal will be 'weight loss' and not 'fat loss' for I use this fat as an energy for the workouts like power walking, running, jump rope and own body weight trains like squats, pushups. Once you have achieved weight loss or partially made good-sized progress—you can start to tone your muscles underneath your love handles. As you burn the fat and increase your metabolism through building muscles, that extra padding will eventually go away.

Reasoning being at home and still have an appetite to shed this excess fat over the oblique region of your torso, then you personally require altogether a different sets of exercises for theirs the first part to get fat and the last part to release it.

Bicycle Crunches

Lie one your back with your knees bent and your hands at the back of your head. Do not clasp your hands together. Grab your abs, lifting your shoulders and upper back off of the ground (don't give jerk to the neck while lifting). Initially don't try hard to lift, with time you will make it. At the same time, move your right elbow towards your left knee so that they meet in the middle of your body. Next, switch your position by bringing your left elbow to your right knee. Continue speedily while still keeping your torso raised up off the ground.

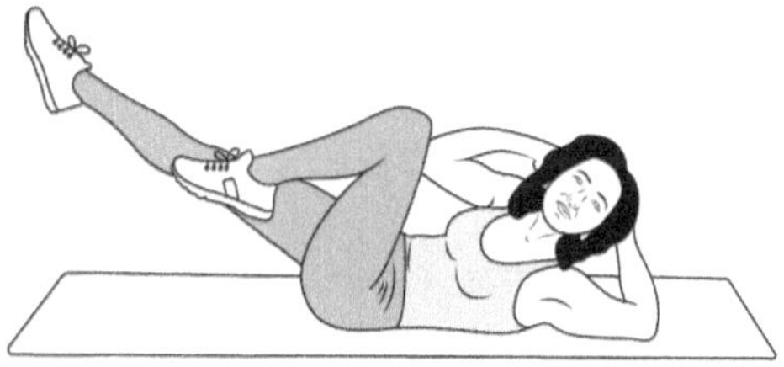

Only being impatient for fixing on any of the part of your body and taking trouble for it may be appealing, but is unwise. Rather, schedule all the exercises during the week for utilising all the muscles of the body, which you ask, I covered in one or the many form of workouts, may perhaps foster to accentuate your aesthetics, additionally to improve your metabolism and, strong bones and …

If in any case, for some reason, you skip this schedule or if you do feel revulsions towards exercise?, which is likeliest with everyone not only you in the long run then, I think, at-least you won't speak for "no" to outstretch your hands, want strongly like a princess and tap your feet to a joyous melody or pulse the rhythmical throbbing of the arteries with the percussion of rhythms of the world; if you talk of me, I do the basic steps of Bharatnatyam holding my hands on my love handles, in this manner this route can be one way for physical fitness, along with mental and emotional stability.

There is a harder and more terrible truth which comes as 'extra calories' form your diet, turns into triglycerides and store them in fat cells around waist. Here I suggest to reduce your calorie intake each day, use unsaturated fats like pumpkin and sesame seeds, flax seeds, nuts (almonds ,hazelnuts, walnuts..) sunflower oil, soybean oil, cold water fish, lean meats, skinned poultry, low-fat dairy.

Also don't encourage your triglycerides to dump around your torso by keeping under control your cortisol and adrenal levels which is raised due to stress and insomnia. Meditate and have a sound sleep.

As long as you eat healthy, drink plenty of water and exercise, I don't endorse specific diet plan for your curvy figure.

Unshapely Hips

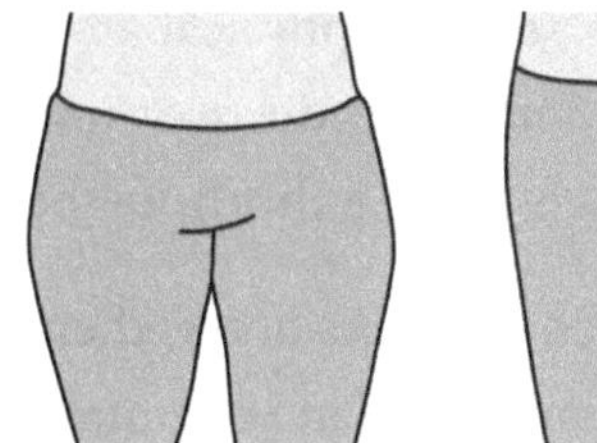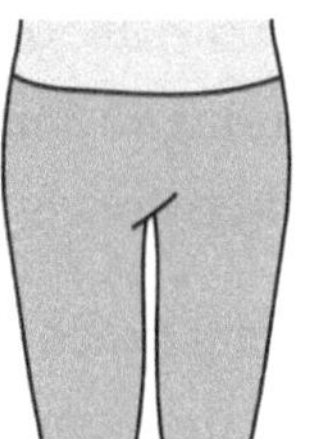

In my hunt with regard to notions about hips as an element of beauty, I got to know hips in different angles and my vision widened when, I saw somewhere from the eyes of photographer who expressed the power of self-expression and individuality by framing the pleasing sensuous curves in his work;

when I read somewhere the poetess personified hips which signifies her unwillingness to be shunted to the side or deemed unimportant by society, and cerebrates her hips as a symbol of womanhood and a source of strength;

and when hips were designed on Kills woven varieties of Turkish flatware rugs where Elibelinde means exactly "hands on hips"; its a motif of a hands-on-hips female figure and their is a genuine belief that it symbolises fertility and motherhood.

Even I'm of the opinion that across the song "hips don't lie", Shakira wants to celebrate womanhood and female empowerment by celebrating her hips.

I comply with the articulation of hips in varied forms that teaches us to keep high regard for your body is capable of rather than feeling loss of face, because you are short of the unjustifiable social standards.

I'm not an exception to those perception. Being a medical person, I sets my sights on disease free long life. My way of praising womanhood is straight through the exigency for rational preventive roadmap of workouts in a way to endeavour the average female functional and aesthetic body (if not standard), that if not achieved, its learnt that, over a period of time might potentially soar our physical and psychological distress. In a nutshell, I am aiming to somewhat delay or reverse some of the changes of ageing which otherwise could be a thorn-in-the-flesh.

Pretty much everyone detest their hips, also the 'hip dips' which were never the problem until you start making a problem. And to my mind hips are now no more the subject of debate.

Of the many questions, I remember the one which one of the freak mailed me several times for the dents in her hips and immediately wanted to fill it.

Look, it has everything to do with your natural anatomy, hip dip is the centripetal recession along the side of your body beneath the hip bone and is due to the scattered fat and muscles in your body structure. They get more or less prominent subject to the width of your hips and the shape of your pelvis.

See, there isn't really a muscle to exercises, so you cant really fill the dents. You can minimise their prominence by maintaining the normal body fat also can develop and strengthen the muscle group around your hips (glutes, outer thigh, inner thigh) for which you can even opt resistance band.

Unlike many factor metabolism is dependent on muscle mass for conversion of calories into energy and one of the secret of building lean muscle mass is in deep hip. Hip-driven exercises increases the metabolic rate, burns your calories faster, relieves pain, improves your ability to move throughout the everyday assignments, also strengthen the hip joint.

To add definition to your hip choose a handful of moves to create a lower body centric routine which includes glutes like lunges, deadlift, hip extensions, step ups; I somewhere discussed in thigh workouts.

And finally, as I always say-aspire for bringing about overall state of health and line up body specific objectives into your workouts.

Complex Thighs

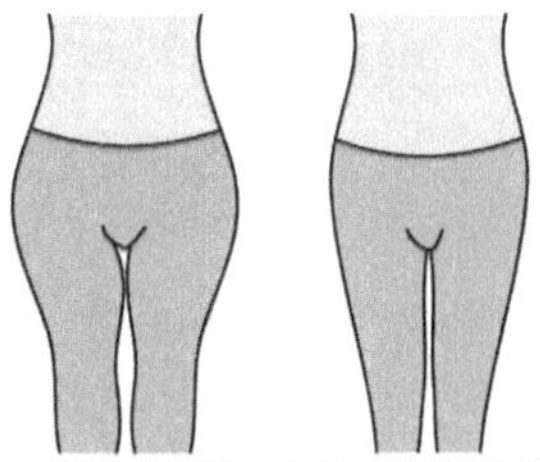

Very often I have seen my patients are open to change, but at the same time are quite stubborn to make a change, just like the stubborn thigh fat who takes a long waiting time to filter this tough break and catch up.

Although, I sympathise with the wage of war and inconvenience of thick thighs leaving you in shambles, at which instant it bumps your BMI, imparts your soreness due to chub rub, makes your spending on jeans futile, and concurrently your vintage dresses thereby decline to adjust you.

Look, thighs are tough nut to crack, although, one and all build castles in the air or fantasise toned and slender thighs, even so we realise that despite of, aimed fat reduction is unfeasible. Optimum within your reach is to tone from the waist and thigh down so it look that way slim and you too can carry your attire boldly.

Apart from fancy to facts, like your upper arm, the upper leg is impressively marshalled like sardines on the front, far and wide obvious in gym as 'quads' entertaining the clubbed sartorious and other four muscles. Although the muscles are nestled in the center, middle, outer below, hidden and crossed diagonal, it bring to mind as one muscle. That's been said because your strength lies in thighs, probably, could be the reason why nerds strangle people (usually lethally) to death with their thighs rather than hands or arms, considering the glory of union of muscles, one way expressing the warm approval for the phrases "unity is strength" and "we are only as strong as we are united, as weak as we are divided".

Fortunately, anyhow we should not see even a bit of further hostilities. This day and age is a point of time for conscious knowledge and implementation of health awareness and well favoured physique, just like today strong legs is meant to enjoy every day activities still pretty pleasing to your eye. I'm trying my hand at both vision, keeping in mind the questionnaire that happen; look for one and the other. I will myself consider as blessed, if even a little for this awareness I begin.

Squats

Since you can bring about while standing up and without extra weights, at first, I recommend squats to sculpts your butt, hips and abs together. For this to start with, you can catch hold of a wall, chair or the edge of the table for support or without it also. Rest, follow the inherent part and call to stand firm against the pull on or push off movement as shown in figure. Aim 3 sets of 12–15 repetitions of this squat. You feel lower back pain if you put your weight on lower back muscles, instead put your weight on your glutes and quadriceps.

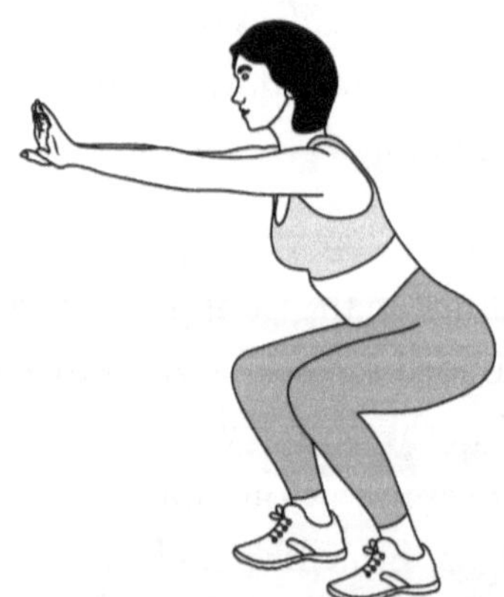

Lunges

When it comes on thighs and the only choice is to get strong, work on both the legs at the same time like lunges do. Standing tall, forward with one foot before your leg reaches to 90. Thereafter, lift your front jumping leg to return to the starting. Repeat 10–12 reps on one leg or you can switch off between legs. You can also do walking lunges to elevate your heart rate.

Do not step too far for it can hurt your knee or you can also loose your balance, also do not step too far back, then you won't get a proper 90-degree bend.

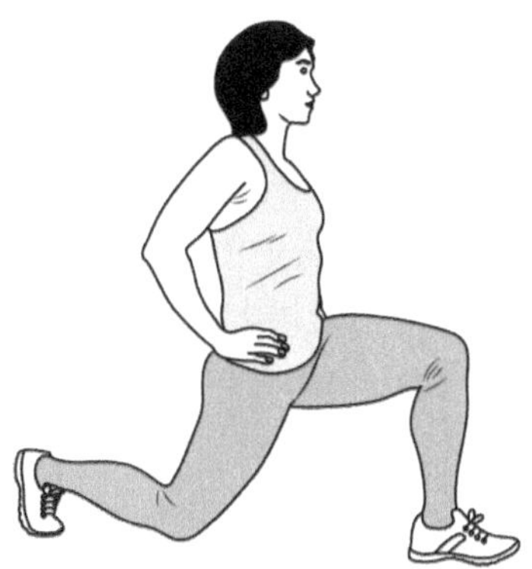

Plank Leg Lifts

If you appropriately conduct your planks, this you could try for next.

Take a plank position, (with shoulders, hips, and ankles in a line) with hands shoulder-width apart. Keeping abs engaged, raise right leg off the floor until its at about hip height. Maintain right foot at the flexed position. Pause at this position and feel the burn. Then lower your right leg back to the floor. Then continue with your left leg. Do these movements alternately with 10 repetitions of each for 3 sets.

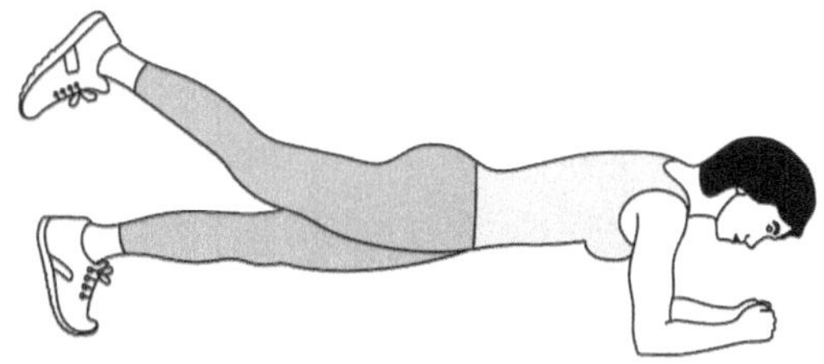

Single Leg Deadlift

To strengthen the entire of your body's posterior kinetic chain, deadlift is pretty much reigns supreme. It is a hip-hinge movement that strengths your legs, back and core, means, it works on all the major muscles. You can do variation by lifting off the ground your one leg and extending out behind you. It requires your stability. The balance and strength obtained from this workout will help your glutei, destroys all traces of nervousness, good for your nerves.

Begin standing with your feet hip-width apart and parallel. Lean forward from hips, shifting your weight onto one leg while your leg engages and starts to extend straight behind you. Form the "T" shape of your body with your hands hanging down. Slowly bring in your extended leg and return to starting position. Repeat with the other leg. You can add some weights to your hanging hands.

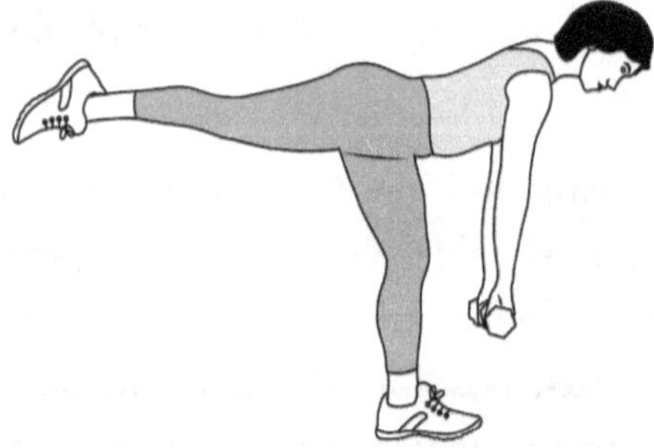

Step-ups

Make repetitive movements of the one legged squats on the raised platform without feeling pressure on your knees. Stand in front of a step or a heavy box. Step the right foot on the box as shown in figure and straighten it, bringing left foot to meet your left so you are standing on the box. Return to the starting position by stepping down with the right foot, then the left. Like this complete 15 steps with right foot, then with left foot. Complete 3 sets.

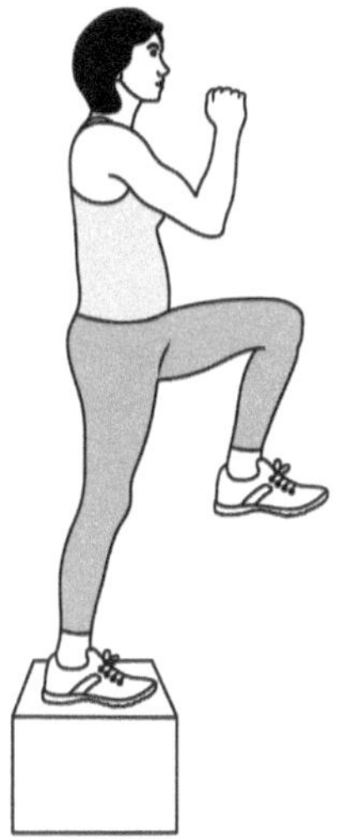

Speed Skater Jumps

This could be one of your aerobics move. It strengthen your heart also.

Start jumping back and forth by crossing your legs behind your arms softly, preferably by small jumps initially thereafter add larger skater jumps and weights.

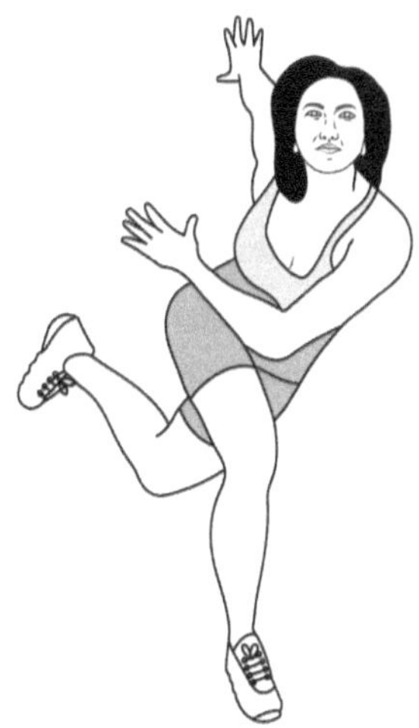

Dead Butt

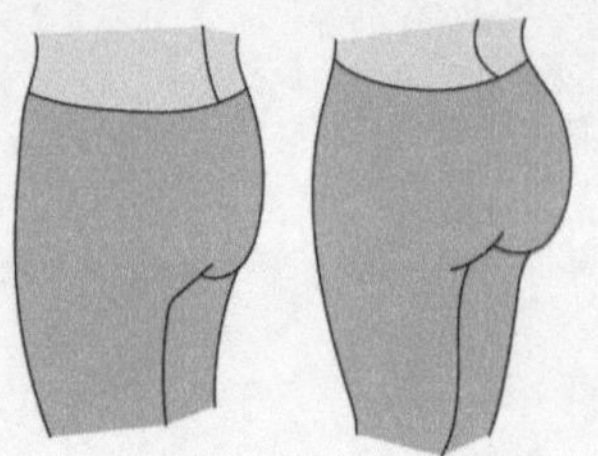

Have you ever heard that equally similar to brain, your butts as well losses its memory and fail to remember its purpose. Or else, make it clear that our bodies are not predetermined for sitting long haul and sitting-around at length suck in buttocks.

Yes, its neurological hang up of butt and it doesn't activate as it used to be. Truth is that the glutes and its brother muscles serves as a foundational structure in our anatomy and if neglected it becomes weak or dead and bring about poor posture, low back pain, balance issues, lack of strength and could potentially increase the risk of injury. It also contribute a top range of health issues- achilles tendonitis, shin splits, runners knee and idiotibial band syndrome.

Ladies think apart, your glutes are the most overlooked area to discuss, possibly because of stupid mindless non acceptance. But, it's the apple of researchers eye to dig foremost on "female butt", a feminine part that has been historically connected to aesthetics across all cultural diversity. Remember, it's the very own area where female can show off as its the numero-uno weapon (our some of strength) where women are generally stronger than men. That's why the girl next door with great bum fascinates more men, it's what Darwinian theory propound.

To the fun side of it, you must have heard "Women's Beautiful Buttocks" contest to "Miss Bum Bum" contest where female turnout to compete each year for "Best Butt" in the country where roundness, curviness and firmness is focused on participants behind. Such, on condition that you as well wish fire up your glutes regularly.

Although 70 percent of our butt is destined by our ancestors, even so for the remaining number you have no choice other than to conquer the under-utilised glutes by lifting and strengthening your butts which otherwise could run short of oestrogen, increases risk for heart problem, depression, weak bones, etc.

Everything has shape. If you look for it, women's butt is no different to that and speaks a lot about her health. So, my solitary purpose is to make you understand your butt shape personally and trigger off the right cause of disfiguring it, furthermore customise your workouts.

1. Square shaped

This butt forms the shape from hip bone to the outer thigh in more or less a straight line. Numerous women have 'hip dips' or 'love handles' with this shape which theorise raised cortisol (stress hormone) and thy lack in ample exercises. Accordingly, harp upon stress relieving meditation and planks.

2. Heart shaped

This shape has tapered waistline and fat is distributed in the lower part of your bottom or thighs. Too big thighs and hips indicates faulty diet, fewer action and stress, which to a degree increases risks of osteoarthritis and cellulite. In that event, stretch out for diet correction, accelerate your activity levels and destress yourself through yoga.

3. Inverted triangle shaped

This shape has a more fullness at the top, near your waistline and ageing makes the fat run to the other parts of the body due to lesser oestrogen, creating less volume in the lower butt cheeks. Declined oestrogen can even lead to heart problems, depression, osteoporosis, risk of urinary tract infections and weight gain. Guard your heart at earliest. During the menopause period, the bone mineral density (BMD) lowers and there is deterioration of bone tissue which makes the bones fragile, or you can say at menopause the normal bone turnover cycle is impaired by oestrogen deficiency, which results in net loss of bone. Add calcium supplements.

4. Round shaped

Represents proportion of full hips and fat is distributed around the butt cheeks including the upper parts. If you want to keep up with this asset, find yourself in the pink only at the expense of fat assembled in the buttocks.

How to check out your glutei weakness

Stand with your hands over your head, palms facing each other. Raise your right foot off the ground and balance. Observe the left side of your hips, if it dips down, its a sign of glutei weakness and suggests your glutei need work. Correspondingly do an attempt on the left side.

Out of many of my favourite exercises, I would like to share the exercises concentrating on the lower part of your body specially the glutei muscles which are extremely important to embrace your curves, create your configuration and have a major impact on your overall body strength.

It's the matter of concern among many whether, when and what time should glutei stretches should be worked out?

Glute stretches should ever can be done, as a part of your warm up before you exercise which get run the blood to these muscles and set them for motion. Further it's far reaching beneficial after workout with regard to boost flexibility, prevent stiffness, also refine your further tasks.

Likewise can be done anytime when majority of you jammed at your desk or watch your shows for hours making them tight.

In the genesis of buttocks, generally the majestic large muscle-gluteus maximus gets the kudos but the determination of medius and minimus is also crucial but usually underestimated and under-utilised leading to dead butt. The workouts given below will work on all of them.

Clamshell with Resistance Band

Specially to warm up the switch off butt at home, I found clamshell that with resistance band more rewarding for its strengthening and firming your whole butt at an affordable price, equally befitting resistance training without gym instruments. I never the less find these bands enjoying moreover for the simple differing job of 'push -pull'.

Place the band around both legs, just above the knees. Lie on one side with knees at 45 degree angle, legs and hips supported. Contract your abdomen muscles to stabilise your core. Keep your feet in contact with one another as you raise your upper knee as high as you can, without moving the hips or pelvis don't allow your lower leg to move off the floor. Pause at the top for a few seconds before returning the top knee to the starting position. Do 15–20 repetitions on each side.

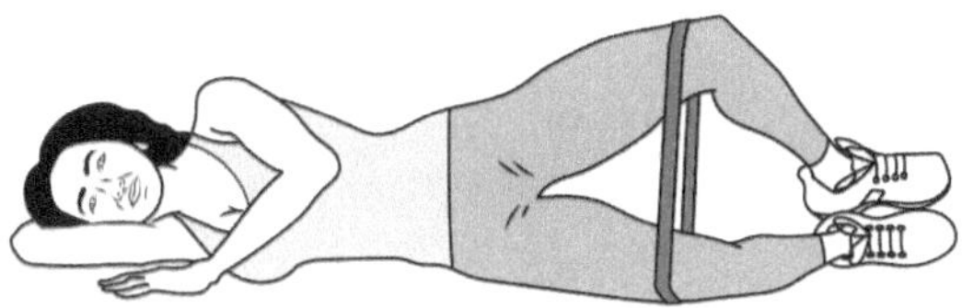

Glutei Bridge with Resistance Band

Be supine on the floor, keep your knees bent; and just above your knees tie the resistance band around your thighs, keep your feet wide apart, and with your hands at your sides and fingers close to the back of each heel. Hold your core so your low back presses against the floor. Push between your feet and lift your hips until they line up with your knees and squeeze your glutei at the top. Lower your hips to the floor to go back to your starting position. Do around 15 repetitions 3 times with a break of 30 seconds in between.

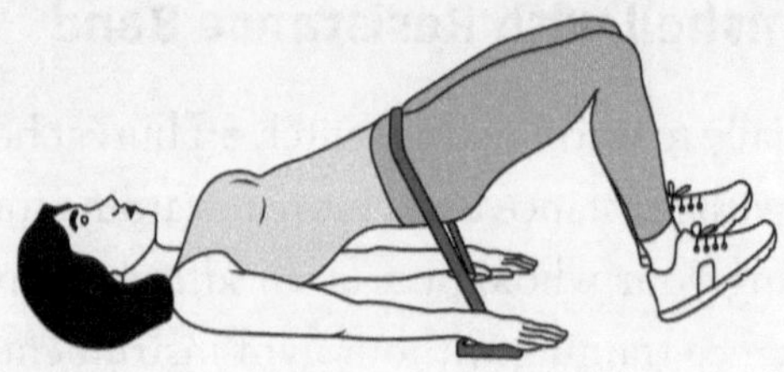

Donkey Kicks

Donkey kicks could be a great relief for those having the desk job for these donkey movements prevents the sedentary hours in chairs and I rate this workout first in isolating the biggest and bulkiest glutei muscle.

Grab the resistance band handles and position your hands so they are directly under your face, elbows bent. Hook your right foot into the band on the other end. keeping your back straight push your right leg out and up. Draw it back into your chest for 1 repetition. Complete 10–15 reps for 2–3 sets on each leg.

If you don't have resistance band, then you can use your own resistance while pushing back your foot toward the ceiling and squeeze butt at the top.

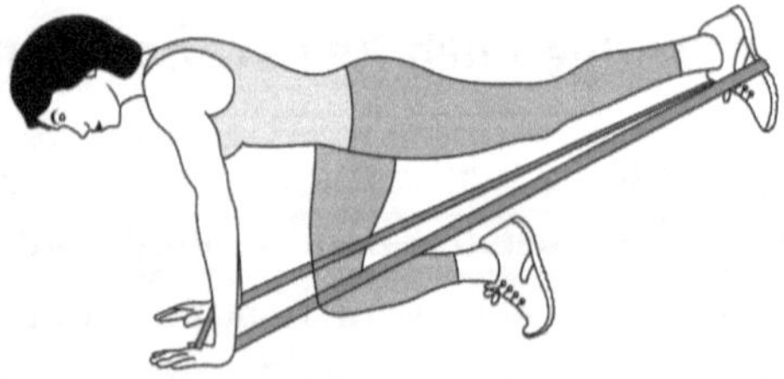

Squats

As I told you earlier beginners can try squats which are great way to build muscles with zero equipment like body weight squat, pile (sumo) squats, pulse squats, jump squats, split squats to make your butt and thighs comparatively smaller, tighter, more toned and compass, but even after 4–5 month you have not noticed big butts, or if you are very lean, means you need to add some weights like goblet squats which would make the muscles grow.

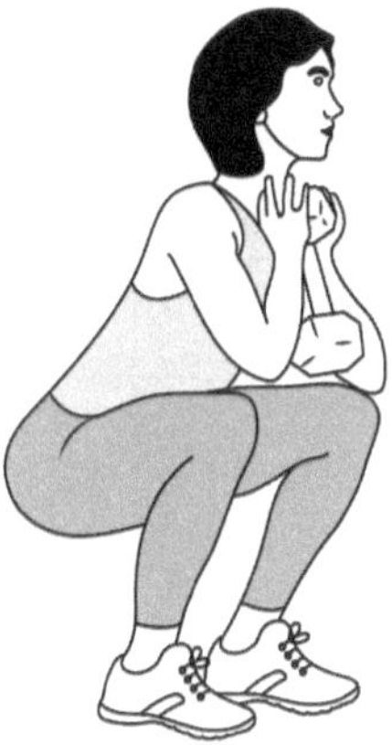

Cardio

If your aim is to loose fat then add regular cardio or high intensity training on most days of the week to lose fat all over.

Glutei Stretches After Workout

Stretching regularly is another way to prevent inactive tight glutes.

After the workout massage your glutei with foam roller to increases the blood flow to the area and for loosening the connective tissue around the muscles to table smooth movement. Slowly roll the foam roller along the length of your gluteal crossing one leg over the other. If you have pain or tenderness, get the tender point while rolling, pause and hold that position for 60 seconds and until pressure/pain is dropped.

Complete some numbers of walk with the resistance band looped around your ankles and hip wide part.

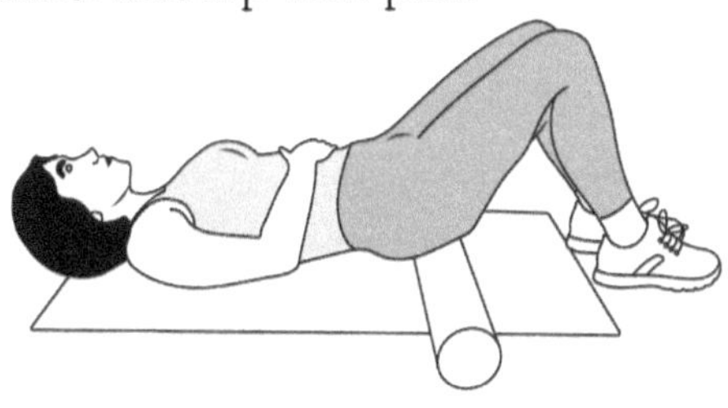

Seated hip abduction with resistance band

Sit on a flat bench with your back straight and your feet on the floor. Hold your hands on the side of the bench near your hips. Put a resistance band around both legs at the knee. In one motion, push your knee away from each other and then push back to touching each other, it should look like your are doing butterfly with your knee.

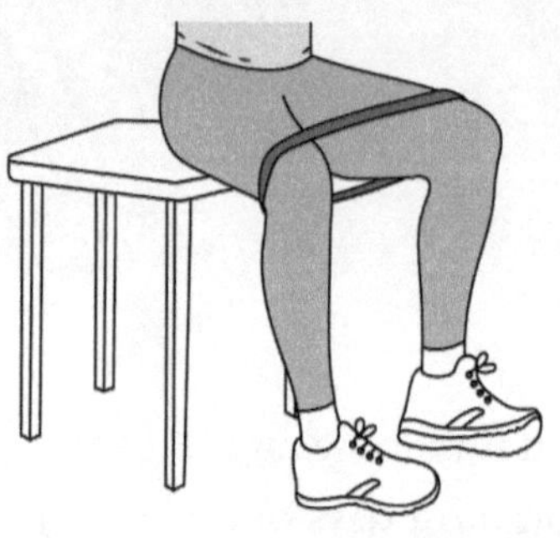

Dimples

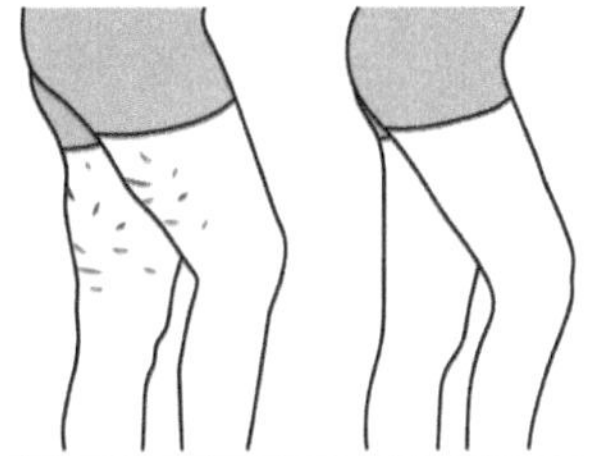

Cellulite is not just a speculation, it's actually a fact of life like wrinkles, stretch marks, freckles and comes as fat in the course of time and accelerates through fibrous band that fasten skin to muscles of the thighs, hips, buttocks; packed in lumps instead of layers giving it a dimpled appearance.

The severity scale of cellulite appears from orange peel as milder to cottage cheese as moderate to mattress appearance as severe. But don't measure its severity, either ask yourself "would these prejudices stop me in their own favour"?

Cellulite wasn't viewed the way today as an unattractive feature or the flaw to be banished. In present time, with dermal fillers pooling, passion for fashion outfits and the gym trend on rise in India, many women see cellulite a body's undesirable feature. Consequently the question of self-esteem or cosmetic issue, glamorous looking is on rise which comprise embracing your rolls and stretches.

But if you are a nonchalant and can't bring yourself to do something, let nature take course of the dented shadows and mushy dimples on your buns, legs and thighs to materialise.

As you see change is inevitable and equivalent. It's been said that about 85% of all women of 21 years and older have cellulite and thighs are more prone due to more fatty tissues and also as age advances or menopause comes the oestrogen flow to the connective tissue under the skin also decreases. Low oxygen results in lower collagen production, poor lymph drainage, poor circulation and fat cells enlarge and beaches noticeable.

Do not rush for the passive and superficial beauty treatments. Remember no one will do your push-ups for you do need to take the steps. Also, you need to be in a positive community and someone to guide you along until you look gorgeous, get your health and energy back.

Don't engage in unusual to find out something you are afraid of, rather we all will stick to the way of workouts we held, which will help to keep it at bay your worries because of its good beneficial reasons.

Foremost, hit your lower body to build crucial muscle foundation below the fat in the area and burn calories. In general, the lower body exercises which I discussed earlier like squats, jump squats, unplug kicks, jumping jacks, lunges or single leg hip raise helps erase some of the butt dimples.

Also other strength training like some weight lifts (with light weight dumbbells, resistance band) or climbing, jumping,… replaces fat with muscles and makes your skin look smoother and firmer. Like this make 2–3 sessions/week of leg and glutei exercises in a way it boosts your metabolism, improves blood flow in your whole body and so the lymph drainage. This metabolism boosting benefits of weight work will not only start to smooth out the orange patty peel on your rear end, also build stronger thigh muscles and tightened skin around thighs.

As you can see, I'm always flexible in giving you the options. If you find the workouts bothersome, and can't bring it to happen then, I think dancing would be the best fat burn activity for you would actually enjoy to improve skin elasticity.

Encourage Circulation

Some believes that cellulite occurs more often in areas with poor circulation. Consistent massage can be promisingly improving your lymphatic drainage by draining excess fluid, re dispersing fat cells, well upholstered skin and can make cellulite less apparent and make you more relaxed.

Exfoliation

Exfoliation is physically scrubbing the skin with an abrasive. I suggest to go for the non chemical exfoliant like microfibre cloths, sugar and salt crystals, sponges, loofahs, brushes for it dehydrates and deflates fat cells and making cellulite look a little obvious and also helps to transit vital nutrients to its cells and do away with other chemical byproducts, that can accumulate in the fat layer for good sized cellulite.

Look, what might work for you would fail for others. But we could at least add some harmless inclusions for which we don't have to rely on investing hefty, expensive lotions, or other captivating propagandas.

Finally, do not make a lack of water in your body as it assists to encourage circulation and lymphatic flow, somewhat minimising one of the cause.

Varicose Vein

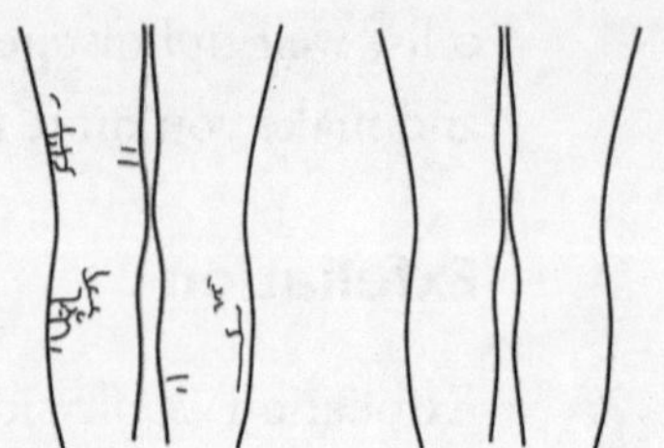

Lockdown was the time prime of divergence from the outside world to confined to the home world. I would say, it was the invent of silent learnings, with limited measures, bounded elbowroom, but we are thankful to our at-hand environment which never left us alone. Their hugs worked as magic for the body and soul in its varies form like sunbeam, unpolluted fresh air or more, what we were going to loose somewhere.

During the pandemic I sought every effort which are likely to bring calmness and immunity amid the disturbed phase of lockdown and there I find ways to use the immediate source of it- the sun rays. To get it, I don't have to go far seeing that it directly falls on my terrace garden. Duly I decided to get in sun trap, tan myself and consequently trigger my brain to release serotonin to boost my mood.

On such leisurely early morning with my sundress, I turned my face to sun and all my shadows fall behind. Also its rightly been said that nothing is hidden in the sun. It happened to me when the rays unexpectedly exposed my hidden varicose veins to my daughter, to her surprise she had to scream in astonishment "mom, there are spider web on your thighs".

........., and I thanked this Sun and lockdown who uncover my network of prominent fine arterioles on my inner thighs. Most often I treat varicose veins, despite that spotting them on my legs stir up my mind to well timed audit of my pregnancies, my weight, my aging and my way of living, although I know varicose veins can be like awfully displeasing. Also almost ten to one, are certainly aware of spider veins which is the sibling of the varicose veins. Although we dislike their arrival they are in no way physically noxious.

Pretty much all the time varicose veins sound off for worry. Threatening misfortunes like pain, swelling, restless leg syndrome, tired aching legs, come about but is infrequent.

In extremely rare cases, untreated varicose veins leads to potentially dangerous deep vein thrombosis or blood clots and ulcers. Here treatment is necessary.

Myths is after all the never-ending story around every ailments. In case of varicose veins the frequently asked myths at my clinic itself demonstrate the outright solution for varicose veins.

1. Is exercise distressing the varicose veins?

Me: Let's debunk this common myth on varicose veins- do not stop exercise for the fear of varicose veins. You can go for hand full of routines, rather you can use low impact exercise like walking, stair climbing, cycling, swimming that helps to move your legs and get the blood flowing without causing excessive pressure and look into gradually easing exercises from the other side into a workout week.

2. I can't do without weights, should I continue it with varicose veins on my thighs?

Me: Yes, you can. But it's better to err on the safer side. Be careful in choosing your workout, shift to lighter weights as heavy weights put the pressure on abdomen and impedes the flow of blood to the heart and collects the venous blood in your leg veins.

Also, wear the stretchy socks (compression stockings) during and after lifting weights. Wearing it puts gentle pressure to your lower legs, maintain blood flow and reduce discomfort and swelling. Remember, promptly go for a walk or gentle stretching after your weight lifts to secure your blood flow again.

A general rule is to exhale as you raise the weights to curl, then simply inhale as you are coming back to your starting position and repeat. This breathing causes movement in your abdomen, which in turn assists the blood flow throughout your body and decreases pressure in your lower leg veins.

Most essential- don't hold your breath during your moves.

3. I'm at higher risk of varicose veins………..?

Me: For me the highest risk a person can take is to do nothing. To make your way along varicose veins, appraise low impact exercises and for hazards avoid or minimise leg lifts, lunges, extended abdominal posturing exercises like squats, sit ups, crunches.

Cut down your salty food and eat vegetables like onions, bell peppers, spinach ,broccoli which contains flavonoids to improve blood circulation.

4. What are the alternatives that can be performed at home during this lockdown?

Me: At home you can boost the identical benefits of running and jogging by walking for at least 5–10 minutes on your terrace or the perimeter of your building after every half an hour and even if that is not possible, march in your place while cooking.

I would suggest to opt for slow jog on softer surface like grass instead of running which would cause serious devastation.

Or to mimic cycling, lie on your back and pedal your legs in the air by drawing your knee towards your chest and giving some self resistance to push forward or, you can ride a stationary bicycle at your home.

For optimal circulation use knee-high compression socks which helps prevent blood from pooling in your lower leg during sitting for long hours, standing, travelling and even during exercise.

Use loose clothings at home and avoid high heels, tight fitting jeans which can cause long lasting negative effects on your tendons and bones.

5. I'm having a physical limitation, how could I continue?

Me: You can rock your feet from toe to heel to keep blood moving into your legs.

For that stand in front of table, chair or any solid object as an aid for support. Rock your weight forward and rise up onto your toes. Stay with this position for 5 seconds. Next, rock your weight backwards onto your heels and lift your toes off the ground. Stay for 5 seconds. Redo the sequence according to your wish.

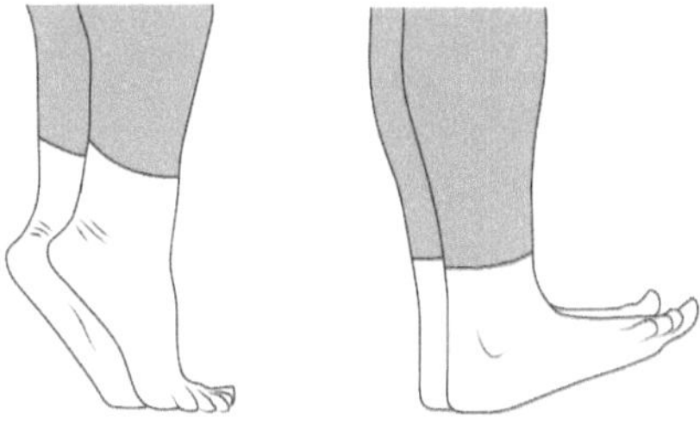

Incontinence

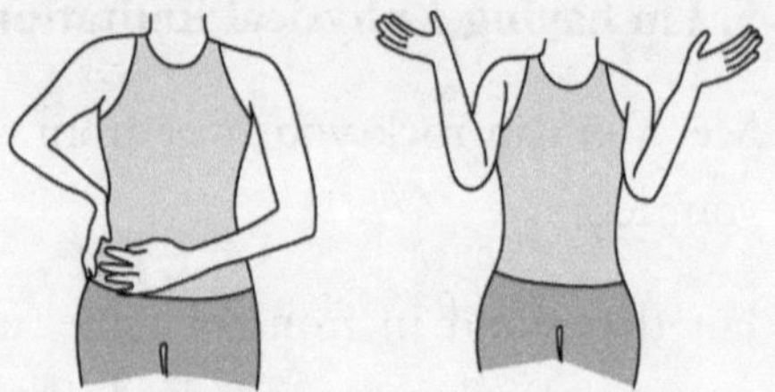

So far, I spotlight the issues of expected aging, but the present concern is not really a coherent fragment of aging yet specifically prevailing over broad scale in elderly.

During the time across the lyrics "suffer in silence" like a shot my phone rang wherefore from a lady who doesn't want to grieve for her go through in silence, which I would say "a silent killer".

And here on this point it made me to differ with the lyrics for to my mind, 'why to go in silence'? where you can keep hold of this inevitable physical misery of 'incontinence' by touching it in good time to fight shyness off this melancholy.

At the height, even we found no specifics to inscribe the subject entirely in texts where incontinence many a time is marked as ban.

Ladies, the things you take it for granted someone else is praying for it. If not you grin and bear this condition, you don't honestly realise the embarrassment that go along with it. In that event you keep away from the get togethers where you would otherwise keep wandering a neighboring lavatory. At this time the gospel truth is that the restrained conduct is more of emotional collapse than the physical encounter.

Incontinence implies that a person urinates when they do not have an urge for. Hear the control over the urinary sphincter or anal sphincter is either lost or weakened.

It occurs when the group of muscles that support bladder, small intestine and rectum in the pelvic floor under sudden, increased pressure(stress), are too weak to hold the urethral sphincters or anal sphincter closed, leading to involuntary leakage of urine during everyday activities such as sneezing, coughing, laughing or exercising, while some gets sudden leakage after the signal of urge. Diseases like chronic constipation, kidney diseases, diabetes, Alzheimer's, Parkinsonism, vascular diseases increases the risk. We have to understand what causes incontinence then you can get it away from embarrassment to some breathing space.

Everything below our chest is supported by our pelvic floor. Pregnancy, excess weight, aging put pressure on the pelvic floor leading to gradual weakening. These muscles additionally contract and expands muscles for defecation, urination, sexual and reproductive function.

Out of the many types of urine leakage, we can think of stress and urge incontinence to control by our efforts. The causes of incontinence are many and its treatment falls into two categories; conservative management with medications, certain devices and surgery while the other category your doctor may recommend you exercises rather than drugs or surgery.

One of my patient speak for the reasons she pick up non specified means and aids in some of the anonymous, not refined magazine, but I strongly disregard it as this problem is not easier than said and should be persuaded thoughtfully right from initially sticking to the protocol of physical examination through specified doctors and thereafter go to, for the causes of incontinence are many and likewise treatment fall. If not counselled for surgery you can opt for the conservative management, bladder training techniques and pelvic floor exercises.

Bladder Training

Bladder training aims to lower the incidences of leakage to avoid frequent bathroom visits and the amount of fluid your bladder can hold.

Maintain your daily bathroom diary and record it, no matter when you have the urge to go, too when you leak. Using this guide, follow the techniques below to help you gain more control over urination.

Delayed Urination

In this technique, learn to put off urination when you feel an urge. Every time you feel the urge, try to hold urine for 5 minutes. When it's to wait for 5minutes try to increase the time for 10 minutes. Continue to increase the amount of time until you are urinating every 3–4 hours.

Scheduled Bathroom Trips

Here, step right to control incontinence by going to bathroom at set times. If you scheduled your time to visit bathroom every hour, gradually increase time upto the limit that works for you.

Relaxation Technique

Is used when you feel the urge to urinate before your scheduled time has arrived. Concentrate on your breathing, slowly and deeply, focus on relaxing all other muscles. If possible, sit down until the sensation passes. Thereafter adhere to the schedule.

Pelvic Floor Exercises

Your gym instructor on prima fascia has a fix to amend the strength of every single muscle of core and the extremities but how about the muscles around the urethral opening (which control urination), vagina and rectum? Here you have to stay off the beaten path to a lesser known Kegel exercise and self assessment.

How to unearth the on-target muscle to exercise?

To avoid the failures of exercises, initially one should be able to trace the right muscles to target. First and foremost, for tracing the muscles of urination, pull in and squeeze the muscles of the pelvic floor by stopping urinating mid stream. The muscles you use to cut off urination are the exact muscles to work on and to tighten.

If you are not sure, do the activity when you out of shame try to stop your passing gas in front of others, or insert the sterile finger into your vagina and tighten the muscles as if you are holding in your urine and then let it go.

Try for long squeezes for three to five seconds then relax for further 3–5 seconds. Frequent practice make them strong and slowly increase the frequency for 20–25 repetitions for 2–3 times/day. Once you have practice for a month or twos, you can do this exercise any time like while sitting or lying down, make it a habit for lifetime.

Squeeze and Release

In addition to Kegel ,try

a. Short contractions - means tighten the fast muscles of the pelvic floor as quickly as possible and release the muscles. Be aware while tightening the muscles, take a deep breath and exhale and think as if you are lifting the muscles upward. Repeat the exercise 10 times and complete a total of 3 sets.

b. long contractions- should last for 10 seconds or hold the contraction of the pelvic floor as long as you could hold it easily.

Caution: ensure to empty your bladder and rectum before exercises.

Pelvic Floor Ball Squeeze

This exercise take part in strengthening your inner thighs and glute muscles thereby intervening with the pelvic floor muscles. Sit up straight in a chair or lie down and place an exercise ball or a firm pillow between your thighs. Squeeze the ball and hold for 10 seconds. Repeat 10 times, this will help out in improving bladder control.

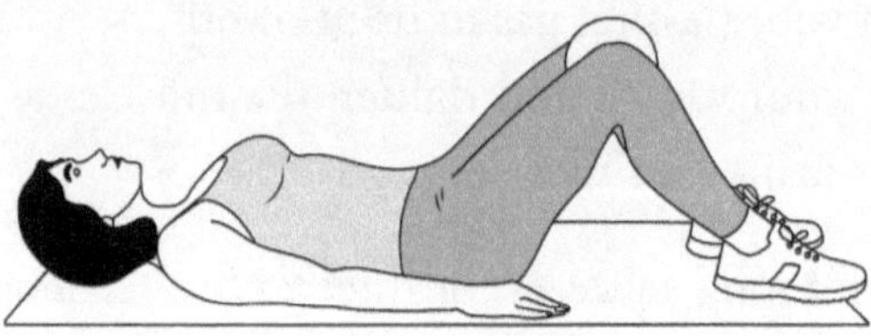

The stretching with resistance band I told you after butt workouts is equally beneficial to strengthen the inner thighs and glute muscles. Here, while pulling your knees away to the sides and bringing them back together, contract your inner thighs and glute muscles and finish one move. Repeat.

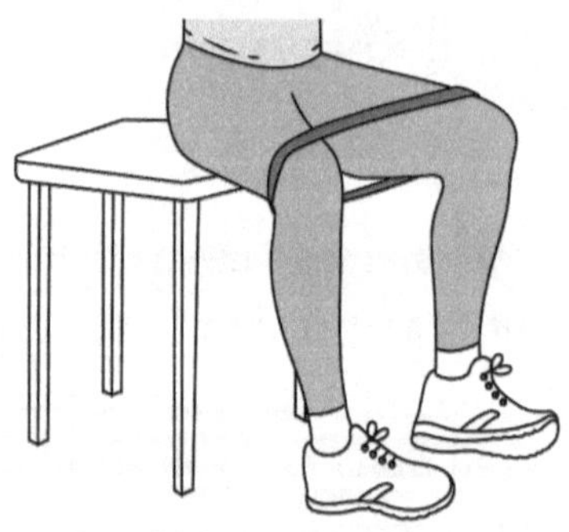

C Curve Abdominal Contraction

It's basically the movement of the spine which strengthen the deep abdominals while stretching the muscles the back

Sit up tall with your legs slightly bent in front of you make a C-shape curve of your body by drawing your abdominal muscles towards your back and with your arms extended. Then straighten your back. Repeat.

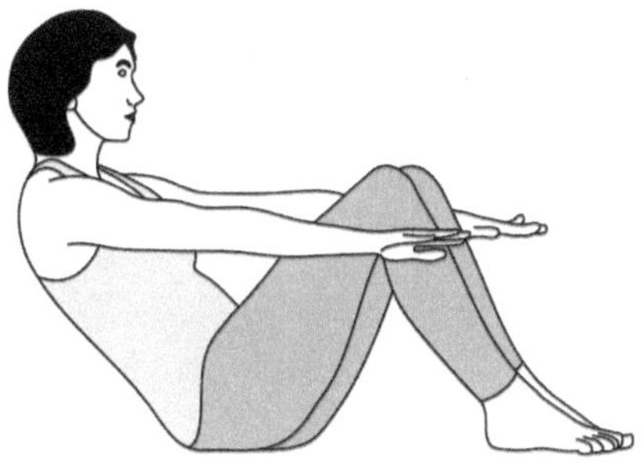

Caution- once you work on weak pelvic floor avoid sit ups, lifting heavy weights in gym, jump and hit.

Bowel Incontinence

Bowel incontinence is caused by the damage to the muscles around the anus (anal sphincters).

Females are affected by accidental bowel leakage twice as male due to damage to the anal sphincters and their nerves while vaginal childbirth and aging. Other potential causes could be from diarrhoea, constipation, inflammatory bowel disease, in cognitive impairment, rectal prolapse, rectal surgery.

Begin a program of regularly contracting the muscles used in urinary flow.

Bowel Training

Schedule bowel movements at the same time each day. This can prevent accidents in between.

Moo to Poo

In the pace of work in the morning, we to get rid of constipated bowel somehow strain the abdominal muscles and deal with it. This weakens your pelvic floor muscles. A simple tactic can rescue you. Also called as

'Brace and Bulge technique' which I discussed further. In this, simply you have to make the "M" and "OO" sounds while sitting wide and bulging your abdomen forward, remaining happens by itself.

Note- Kegel aren't for everyone, if your pelvic floor muscles are always tight these exercises can do more harm than good.

Uterine Prolapse

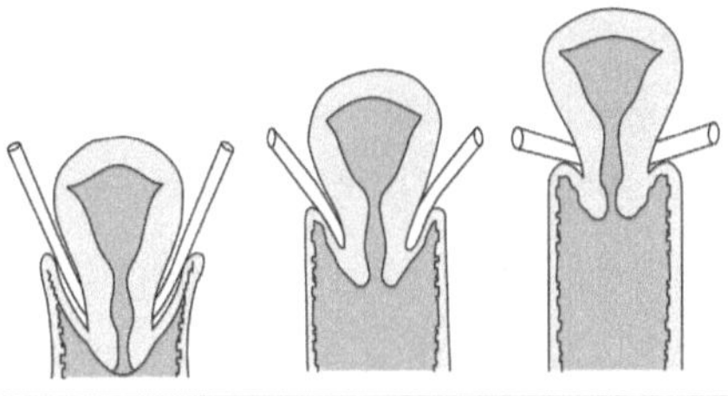

Whoa, gravity stay the hell away from me

Whoa, gravity has taken better men than me

Now how can that be?

Just keep where the light is.

Come on keep me where the light is.

I pursue poems for the reason that it hypothesises the prospects of hope in the dawn of life and serves as motivation to bear down trauma when the situation is grave.

In the perspective, attempting to derive speculations from the poem "Gravity" written by John, the best I can palpate is John's concerned about growing up and older, as a further matter for the burden of living the life of excuses.

Also, the line "come on keep me where the light is" seems a call for the right timely help aiming the unavoidable for whom we are not yet upto to counteract gravity, ageing and times hardship on our bodies.

John is using "Gravity" as a metaphor for aging and fear of. This fear is equally anticipated even in the face of aging in women and I might blame it on "Gravity".

From the aggregate of my entire wide range of subject matters, you must have got to know the crux of my writing "Aging Gracefully", where it revolves around gravity as a synonym for aging in the nature of droops, slippage, fall; since gravity is not only responsible for many of the large scale structures in the universe, also for our necessary body functions under its presence.

The different individuals of the same species verbalise heart as glorious at the point they own no way judge uterus. In a way, women have to her owns name the ownership of brain and uterus carrying out chores as a mother and congresswomen despite of obstacles and hardships, but as we know, she find lack of choices or zero options when it comes to her achy uterus, silent cries and nightmares, to resist or cease her pains, weakening and breakdown.

Every women body change and experience the pull of gravity over time, but I sense, the most prone place is our vaginal support and when the vaginal support weaken or break down, is called "vaginal prolapse" or "pelvic organ prolapse".

Each of us women experience some degree of prolapse but some are more susceptible like who have had multiple vaginal birth, other experiences can also lead to prolapse like constipation, menopause, pelvic surgeries, chronic cough, heavy lift jobs.

Here, bit by bit the uterus slips (also the bladder or bowel) into the vagina, to begin with its upper half, then plunge nearly to its opening, at a greater distance uterus protrudes out of vagina and eventually becomes apparent.

During the process women manifests sensation of heaviness and pressure in vagina, constipation, painful sexual Intercourse, some pop up low back pain that eases when lying down.

I think, most of us are not far from the above reasons which are sure to crop up after a time frame. Hence looking at the severity and complications, it's imperative to seek professional help.

To be specific, in the initial two stages Kegel exercises and other pelvic floor exercises do favour and sometimes also prevent the organs from slipping down further. However its mandatory to get familiarise with the muscles around vagina, urethra, anus and do it rightly what instructed and if not restricted by your doctor, I suggest everyone to get ready for strengthening the muscles of pelvic floor, ageless. Under normal conditions also they don't have any bad influence. In my entire gym, not one notice my Kegals act when I do it with leg raises lying flat surface.

Likewise, It also depends on the act how you carry yourself to relax your pelvic floor muscles including to fight shy of pressuring or straining when urinating and getting bowel movement, make room for learning to relax the muscles in the pelvic floor area such as warm bath just under the body temperature (92–98), some recreation would also help.

In avoiding the evil, we opt for strengthening the abdominal muscle, which is well known to hold the slippage of uterus upto some extent, but should be cautious while finding the right workout, otherwise it would be- in avoiding the evil, we fall for another. Avoid squatting, strong abdomen exercises like sit-ups, core plank or you can keep clear pelvic floor loading by simply reducing the number of repetitions, avoid over bracing the abdominal muscles and make some minor changes in the intensity of abdominal exercises.

As reported, postpartum negligence is one of the top cause for prolapse over time, in India, although postpartum body massage is being carry out for some time as a custom or habitual patronage which in a way helps the tired body muscles to revitalise and get mental relaxation, but actual territory used during delivery is the pelvic floor muscles which needs strengthening. I request every woman or the government, irrespective of the social status, in keeping with your resources, to equally incorporate specifically pelvic floor exercises as an intrinsic program to address muscle weakness and imbalance which otherwise could lead to pain, dysfunction and in the future- prolapse.

Rectal Prolapse

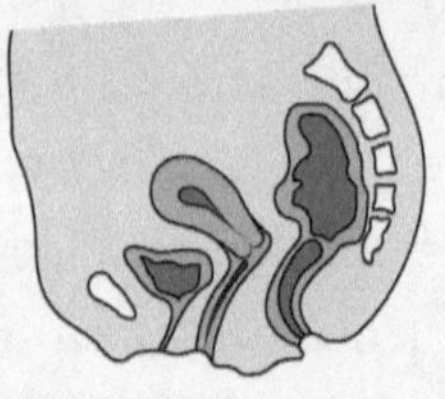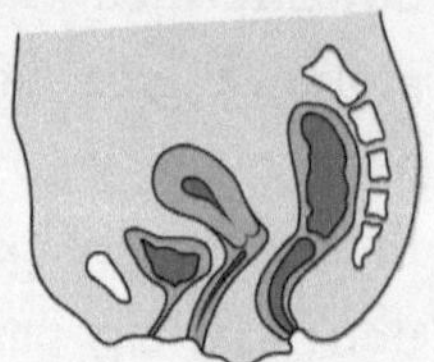

After my graduation, for my immediate internship I was posted at a nearby Primary Health Centre. At the time examining an old lady, she was skeptical about mentioning her symptoms and from her body kinesis I opt for the local examination of lower orifice. Just when I positioned her on the inspection table, I stayed stunned to notice a red fleshy mass out of her rectum with infected foci and to so much of degree, such I didn't get to see ever during my clinical postings. And double to my surprise, even in this perilous condition she was static with poker face as if she has to swallow the absolute truth.

In practical terms, women neglect themselves to deport their domestic and external responsibilities and turn vulnerable in a way that puts their health, safety or well being at risk.

Here, again I remember the words "why to bear in silence? ….".

The spectacle of rectal prolapse goes either in terms of partial when the rectal mucosa stick out of the anus, or complete when the rectal wall protrudes … and even seen as intersusception when eventually it collapses but stays inside and does not come out.As a result, stool may leek uncognizably from anus, also mucus, or blood leaks. Also, you can find an abiding feeling of full bowel, constipation, you may pass small stools, may get a feeling of sitting on a ball, uncontrolled flatus, or anal irritation including pain, itch and bleeding.

If not for the grave up condition we can try for the initial stage of prolapse.

To avoid these untoward situations, perform the best possible pelvic floor strength and support by foremost digging out the pelvic floor muscles for rectal prolapse, exercise it, further train your pelvic floor muscles for everyday activities. Remember, while working on pelvic floor muscles don't fatigue the muscles .

Initially try lying down and imagine that you are trying to stop wind from passing from your bowel and urine passing from the urethra. Slowly lift and squeeze the muscles in and around the anus, vagina and urethra. let your buttocks and thighs stay relaxed and continue breathing, thereafter relax the muscles in and around anus. You can gradually increase your time length and strength for contraction of muscles.

For strengthening, lift and squeeze them for up to 10 seconds at a time. Relax. Repeat for 10 times in a row.

Later apply brisk strong technique of lifting and squeezing for until 10 times, upto 3 times a day

Train pelvic floor muscles for your everyday activities like upright position, cough, sneeze, lifts and when you sense an urgent desire and need to empty your bladder or bowel.

If you are looking for other exercises in prolapse, try low impact exercise with light weights but, as I said earlier, avoid sit ups, plank, pilates, which increase downward pressure on pelvic floor.

Also, one condition which should not be overlooked is 'rectocele', that condition is only found in women where the muscular walls of the vagina are weak allowing the rectum to bulge and protrude onto vagina and in case of larger rectocele, it build the symptoms similar to rectal prolapse. From some of the case studies, while checking out the questionnaire for causes and symptoms of rectocele, I spotted some women marked the option that while defecating they make use of finger for pressing on the rectocele to pass the stool and thus somehow manage to leave the moment. My question is, nevertheless, upto what extend will you continue? gradually this condition will also start becoming problematic and some time it will also be alienated.

Also for some this is such a condition, what we don't know, unless we go to the doctor for some reasons where the rectal examination is mandatory. One thing is for sure, from among the entire symptoms, that for the period of an entire day woman pays attention to her obstructed defecation.

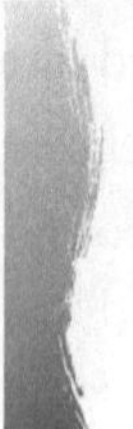

Thus, despite of let it happen to you, take charge of the unavoidable by introducing the self-care measures into your way of life.

For this reason, to help women for emptying their bowel and avoid straining forcefully, Brace and Bulge bowel emptying technique could be the way for primary-care.

Brace and Bulge

When you get an appropriate urge to empty, position yourself sitting correctly on the toilet. How soon are you, first relax your pelvic floor muscles by performing 5–6 relaxed deep diaphramatic breathing exercises. Remember after leaning forward, here you have to make use of tummy muscles to strain and do not strain your muscles in your back passage.

Make your waist wide and bulge your lower abdomen forward which helps to relax the circular muscles around anus to open your anal sphincter allowing you to empty. Make the "M" and "OO" sound where and as stated earlier. When you have emptied your bowel lift and squeeze your pelvic floor muscles.

Obey the Urge

You might think that you are the assemblage of good habits, but while serving for good habits, you may develop a bad habit of holding your poops, although occasionally is not harmful. But very often can lead to constipation and every now and then it may stop your urge to poop, eventually leading to fecal incontinence. Here training your body is about consistency, and if each day you hit the toilet at the same time, is one more step towards your good habits.

Oops! Fart?

……, home is where the fart is, and what if you are not at home, somewhere in gathering. You yourself could think. So before planning to go and also otherwise, avoid gas producing foods like carbonated drinks, some beans, cruciferous vegetables-cabbage, broccoli, cauliflower. Or, come let us fart in the home.

Pump Bump

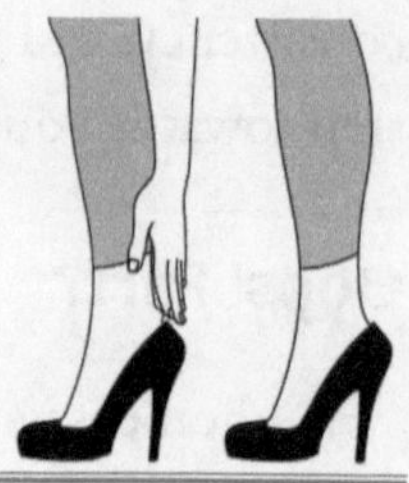

Heels is women skilful passion to bring grace in her body, flaunt in ceremonies, shows and to shine in hip-hop like Beyonce who manages to dance in those stilettos without tripping, else evermore believed to enhance the feminity, as the aftermath of heels was to magnify some sex specific ins and outs of female gait drawing attention, including her swing due to distinguishable pelvic rotations and shorter march.

The world of heels fascinates for good or bad calls for question, but todays women have made up their minds to cling to it whatever the consequences. If you ask me, while prioritising style, beauty and sexiness, aim your high heels something comfortable as they can be, otherwise heels are pleasures with pain.

The term pump bump come after in time doctors observed that women who wear high heels pump shoes had the obstacle in walking and comes as mid to severe pain in the back of the heel when walking, bump is seen at the back of the heel, it swells or get red, calluses or bursitis on the heel are seen where the bump rubs against the shoes.

In fact, the term is used in the context of especially teenagers and young women, I gather that it signifies all women in the race who love dearly high heels and egg heels on for hours.

According to doctors, if the condition is non- surgical, you can arrange for optional. Even if these alternatives cannot rework on your bone or foot structures, can act as an analgesic and better comfort.

If the heel is aching or swelled, you can use ice to relieve. To the matter of utmost importance, avoid rigid back shoes, use heel pads inside the back of the shoes to reduce irritation and friction.

Do stretching exercises to alleviate tension in tight achellis tendon. Like-

Standing Heel Raises

This you can do while standing and steady your weight on the balls off your feet. Carefully raise yourself up onto your toes (as shown in figure) and hold a "tip -toe" position for several seconds then lower yourself back onto the ground.

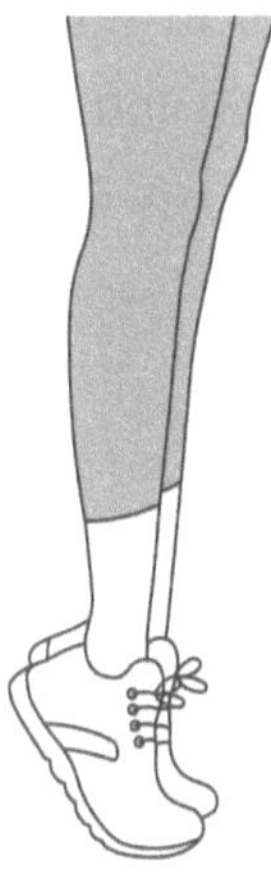

Calf Stretch

To improve flexibility and increase calf strength-

Stand close to the wall with one foot ahead of other, leading knee slight bent. lean toward the wall with your back straight and heels touching the ground, till you feel the stretch in your back leg calf.

Hold the stretch for few seconds. Shift another leg. Go for 10–20 repetitions alternately with both legs for 3 sets.

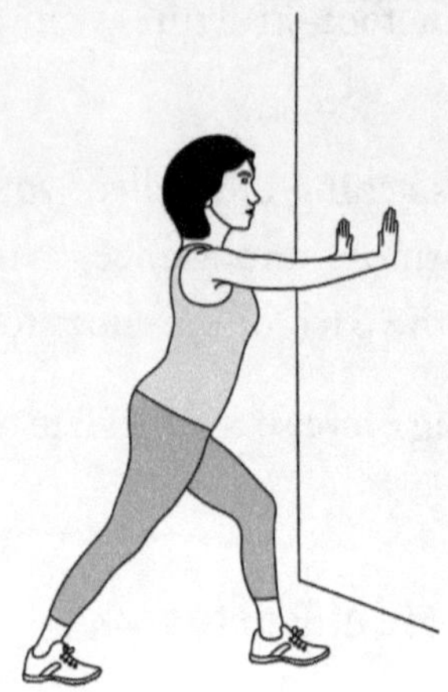

Bilateral Heel Drop

For this workout, take an aid or assistance to balance yourself and stand with your forward foot on the stair and the heels away. Steadily lift your heels and thereafter bring them down as shown in figure upto the level you can achieve. Go for 20—30 repetitions.

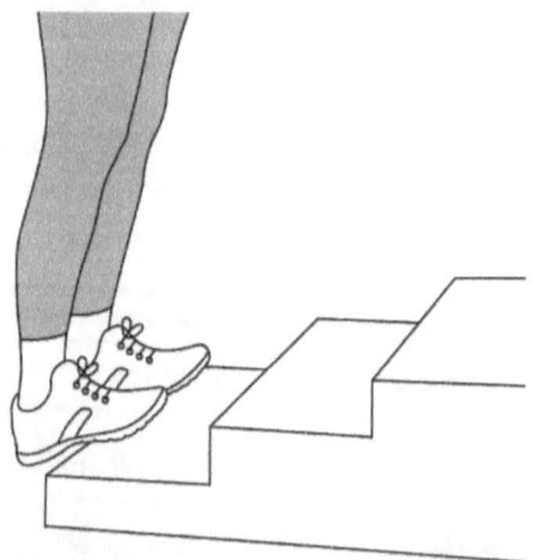

Towel Stretches

Towel stretches stretch the planter fascia on the bottom of your foot.

Sit on the ground with the both legs extended in front of you. Hold with a towel or an exercise band and loop it encircling one foot, clasp one end in both hands.

Kindly back off the towel to pull the ball of your foot towards the body, till you feel the slight tightness in the back of your calf. Hold for few seconds. Repeat with another foot.

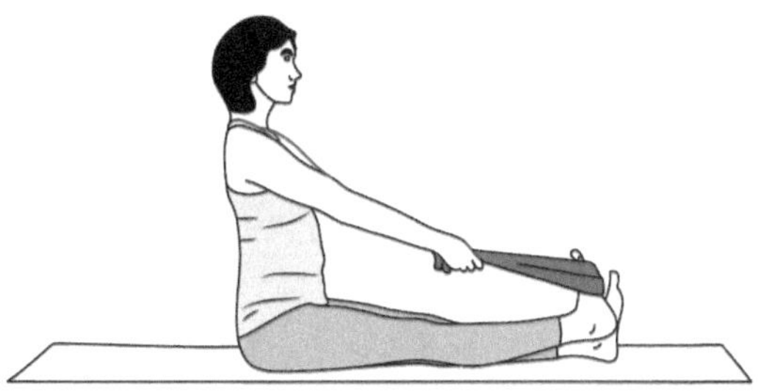

Circumspect while doing strenuous exercises, such as running. Take a gradual approach to avoid worn out injuries.

You may keep aside my book after reading, but don't keep aside exercising. And whenever we meet I will be glad to see how gracefully you are aging.